EVERYDAY WELLNESS

EVERYDAY WELLNESS

12 STEPS
TO
A HEALTHIER
HAPPIER YOU

MaryRuth Ghiyam
with Sarah Durand

ONE PLACE. MANY STORIES

HQ
An imprint of HarperCollins*Publishers* Ltd
1 London Bridge Street
London SE1 9GF

www.harpercollins.co.uk

HarperCollins*Publishers* 1st Floor, Watermarque Building,
Ringsend Road, Dublin 4, Ireland

First published in Great Britain by
HQ, an imprint of HarperCollins*Publishers* Ltd 2020
First published in the United States by HarperCollins Publishers, 195 Broadway,
New York, NY 10007

Text Copyright © MaryRuth Ghiyam 2021

ISBN 978-0-00-842427-5

Printed and bound in Great Britain by CPI Group (UK) Ltd, Croydon CR0 4YY

MIX
Paper from
responsible sources
FSC™ C007454

This book is produced from independently certified FSC™ paper
to ensure responsible forest management.

For more information visit: www.harpercollins.co.uk/green

Designed by Kris Tobiassen of Matchbook Digital

Illustrations on pages i and iii: Faceout Studio

Illustrations on pages vi–viii, 23, 43, 67, 89, 113, 135, 157, 179, 201, 223, 245, and 267:
Crystal Chow

Illustrations on pages 7, 16, 26, 34, 52, 61, 62, 74, 86, 106, 115, 124, 131, 142, 161, 184–85,
205, 210, 215, 231, 250, and 279: iStock

To my mom,
who literally showed me,
by strong and loving example,
how to move forward every day

and

to my father, Richard; my brother, Daniel;
my husband, David; and my children,
Ethan, Elliot, Jacob, and Grace

CONTENTS

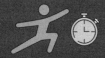
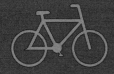

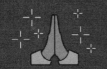

MARY RUTH'S®

THE ART OF HEALTH FOR BUSY PEOPLE

1. **Liquids till Lunch**

Eat three small meals a day, at the anchor times of noon, 3 p.m., and 7 p.m. Make sure to hit all three anchor times!

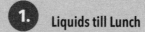

2. **Chew Your Food Until It Becomes Liquid**

3. **Drink Half Your Body Weight in Ounces of Water**

For example: a person who weighs 120 lbs. would drink 60 oz. of water.

4. **Portion Control**

5. **Eat Healthy Foods**

6. **Get Fifteen Minutes of Direct Sunshine Each Day**

Vitamin D is crucial for the mind and body!

7. **Sleep Seven to Eight Hours**

8. **Fifteen Minutes of Stretching**

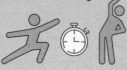

9. **Thirty Minutes of Exercise Daily**

Walking, jogging, elliptical, or yoga. Whatever will get you moving for thirty minutes.

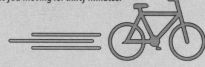

10. **Stress Less**

High stress means higher cortisol levels, which creates cellular damage.

11. **Think Positively**

Use positive thoughts to imbue your day with gratitude.

12. **Believe in a Universal Force of Goodness**

It doesn't matter what you call that universal force–God, Creator–it just matters that you believe that the universe wants the best for you.

Introduction

Moving forward through the chaos and uncertainty that exists in this world can be *so* challenging. Or your day-to-day might be difficult even when you don't have any real struggles. You could be about to enter a great new phase in your life, but its fast pace and tricky challenges force you to work hard and develop true self-mastery.

Whether your situation in life is wonderful or awful, it's easy to feel paralyzed or scared if you don't have a road map, can't summon your power, or worry you might fail or fall behind. When you're faced with a hurdle to clear or a mountain to climb, you might be tempted to crawl into your bed, turn on the TV, and stay there forever. But you can't. You're worth more than that. Your life can be so much better than that, so you *must* get out there and make great things happen.

I have some fantastic news for you. You don't have to conquer all your challenges in one day. You also don't have to be rich, have a fancy degree, or have loads of free time to come out

1

on top. To feel happy, accomplished, fulfilled, or like you're putting good out into the world, all you need are a few daily fundamentals that will help you gain momentum, operate to your highest-functioning degree, and move forward to whatever your goal or purpose is.

It's all easier than you think. You just need to boil the process of moving forward down to the essentials. The actions that will allow you to dislodge yourself from whatever's slowing you down or dimming your energy are as basic and straightforward as taking your daily vitamins.

I can show you how.

When I was twelve, my beloved forty-two-year-old dad died suddenly of a heart condition we didn't know he had. My dad ran our family business and, my whole life, I'd never known a weekday when Richard P. Boehmer hadn't been pacing around the house scratching notes about work on a yellow legal pad with a red pen. On weekends, he and my mom got up early and loved to play golf together. He was always buzzing, chasing, and dreaming . . . and then he was gone. Our house was very, very quiet after that.

I'm the classic oldest child—organized, driven, and focused—and my dad always pushed me to hold my chin up, be a leader, and succeed. After he died, I assumed that going to school, making good grades, and getting into the right college would be enough to help me recover. I did all those things on top of helping my mom around the house, nurturing my younger brother, Daniel, and acting as a shining example of strength and courage for my family. I was just putting one foot in front of the other, though, not thriving. To top it off, I was *crushed* by grief.

When I was twenty, I came home from college for Easter break and was in my bedroom when I heard my mom screaming at the top of her lungs. I ran out of my room and saw her in my seventeen-year-old brother's bedroom, standing above his motionless body on the bed. Then I watched her drag him to the floor and start to give him CPR. But it was too late. He was dead, clutching a phone he'd been trying to use to call for help. We didn't know it, but Daniel had developed a heart condition called *hypertrophic cardiomyopathy*. Suddenly, the hole in my chest that I thought the passage of time had helped heal opened up again, and now the wound was even bigger. My brother had been my best friend. Daniel came to all my basketball games in high school. He made me countless playlists of the best songs to listen to, and he made me laugh about everything, especially during our summer vacations on the Jersey Shore or at Lake Nebo in Upstate New York.

I knew I had to keep going, though, so I went back to college soon after the funeral and worked as hard as I could to prepare for my final exams. I studied abroad in Italy that summer, and when I got back to school, I focused on graduating on time with the rest of my class. If I could succeed, wasn't I living my best life?

Just over a year later, my mom went to the doctor to talk about the right-side facial spasms she'd been having, and she left with a diagnosis of two brain tumors. When she told me, I went numb. *My entire family is going to die,* I thought. *I'm twenty-one, and I'm going to be the last one left.* I didn't feel cursed or unlucky; my pain was physical, like a two-ton weight was sitting on my chest.

My mom endured one painful craniotomy surgery followed by another seventeen months later. Luckily, doctors determined that both brain tumors were benign, but the part of her brain that controls motor function had been damaged during the second operation, and she became partially paralyzed on her right side. During her long months of rehabilitation, I drove home on the weekends to help take care of her. It wasn't always easy but being present for my mom taught me I had a greater purpose: I wanted to help people live healthier, more fulfilling lives.

I went back to school and earned certifications as a health educator and professional business coach. I loved being a student again and I dove into research, soaking up everything I could about health, healing, and the human body. The benefits of healthy food, exercise, alternative therapies, and fasting fascinated me; the interconnectivity of negative emotions and chronic pain opened my mind and showed me things I'd never thought of. I applied all this knowledge—and so much more—to nursing my mom back from her paralysis and into "normal" life. It was the best unpaid job I could imagine, and waking up in the morning knowing I could make a difference for someone I loved was thrilling.

Life was moving forward, and my mom was getting better. We 100 percent believed the worst was behind us and that nothing as bad could happen to us again. Then, in late 2008, Lehman Brothers crumbled, the housing market collapsed, and the Great Recession exploded like an atom bomb. Our family's lumber business plummeted and, over the course of the next two years, my mom had to shut down five locations and lay off 250 employees. She sold our house at a 50 percent loss, borrowed money from friends and family, and started living off credit cards. Within a few years, she was a whopping $700,000 in debt. It was technically her debt, not mine, but we were family, and we were sticking together through thick and thin.

If you've carried significant personal debt, you know how hopeless it can feel. I carried around the weight of that debt in my bones, and every day I woke up tired. But then I jumped out of bed with a smile on my face, went to my job as a Manhattan real estate agent working with my mom, made good money, and surpassed all my company's earning benchmarks. After writing our rent check and buying groceries, we gave every last cent of our paychecks to the debt-management program my mom and I had enrolled in. Then I went back to work trying to sell more, network more, and earn more. I felt like Sisyphus, pushing a boulder up a mountain all day long only to have it fall back on top of me when the sun went down. Sure, I was putting one foot in front of the other, but I was getting *nowhere*. I liked my job, but I didn't love it. And without real fulfillment, I knew my mom and I would never do more than tread water.

This is it, I told myself. *I've had it rough for a lot of years, but this is rock bottom. Time to move forward.*

I put my neck on the line, quit my job, and bought an ad on Facebook that offered free fifty-minute nutritional consultations. I'd developed a simple, free, complete system to help people lose weight, overcome pain, develop better energy, and improve overall health, and my plan was to prescribe it to my future clients, then get them to sign up for a three- to six-month program. I knew I had the tools, advice, and program to help people heal physically, spiritually, and emotionally, and I was more than ready to share them. When my ad went live, I moved my office into a small space in Midtown Manhattan on 47th and Third, waited for the phone to ring, and began doing consultations.

Things were really tough at first. I worked from 9 a.m. till 11 p.m. every day and didn't pay the rent on my apartment for five months. In 2013, I got married on a shoestring, and a few months later I had a miscarriage while I was at work waiting for a client. I still met with them because I was terrified that if I canceled their session, I'd lose the $250 we desperately needed to buy groceries that week. Slowly, day by day, I moved forward, and life started to get better as I chipped away at our debt. Within a year I had eighty to a hundred private clients and was signing up about twenty new ones a month. Best of all, I was happier than I'd been in years. I texted my clients all day long, not just because I wanted to check up on them, but because I truly, deeply cared about them.

I covered *everything* related to health and nutrition. How to lose weight. How to have more energy. How to build lean muscle. How to sleep better. How to let go of addictions and bad habits.

My clients were successful individuals who came from the fields of finance, fashion, media, real estate, and more. Even though many of them had access to the best treatments and the most elite professionals—aestheticians, integrative doctors, cryotherapy, ozone therapy, salt tanks, you name it—they couldn't devote hours a day to their well-being because they were so busy with their careers.

Luckily, I kept things simple for them. My program directed my clients to implement twelve small behavioral changes rooted in foundational health principles into their routines every day. When they learned how to master them, they immediately felt better, developed more energy, and achieved balance. Their health moved forward—and then their lives moved forward—despite whatever obstacles they faced. These twelve actions improved them at the cellular level, which allowed them to operate at their highest-functioning degree. They started to find it easier to self-regulate, modify behaviors, enact change, get out of their emotional ruts, and take their lives to the next level. Each of my clients found the twelve actions basic and doable, yet they uncovered fundamental concepts that were profound and life changing. Best of all, these concepts helped them achieve results that were nothing short of miraculous. They got promotions. They increased their salaries. They married the loves of their lives. They overcame addictions and illnesses and challenges that were standing in the way of happiness and health.

What was fascinating about my clients, though, is that the things that improved their lives the most weren't the expensive regimens or protocols in which they indulged. Instead, their health and happiness took root and blossomed because they used the free, accessible, and universal tools I offer in this book.

A Program of Micro Actions That Leads to Macro Change

My program covers basic health principles that you can tackle within a twenty-four-hour period. Each of the twelve actions is rooted in self-care, allowing you to focus back on yourself and your healing process. The actions may seem small, but they hold the key to making big changes. As you integrate them into your daily routine, everything from your digestion to mental clarity to sleep to immunity improves, giving you an overall feeling of well-being. This better sense of self permits you to function at a higher degree, helping you harness the power to tackle any obstacle life puts in your way.

I'm goal oriented, and if you're reading this book, you probably are, too. Your goals don't have to be huge to get something from my program. When I was in the throes of grief and loss after the death of my brother and during my mom's financial collapse, the twelve actions allowed me temporary freedom from pain. That little bit of momentum allowed me to move forward. A therapist I saw after my brother died backed up this notion for me.

"What's your definition of happiness?" I asked her, searching for something she could point to that would take away the hollow feeling in my gut.

"Satisfaction and happiness are different," she answered. "Satisfaction implies that you're fulfilled, so you don't really need more of anything to feel okay. Happiness is having some moments in your day that *are* happy, even if there are a lot that are sad. But these happy moments stand out, then illuminate and inform whatever the path to your life purpose is."

Let me give you an example. Immediately after my brother died, I was prepared to encounter the kind of pain I'd known when my dad passed away. I braced myself for an onslaught of soul-level pain: a wound that cuts on the spiritual level, affecting every action from the moment of injury forward. Some people say that kind of hurt only happens when someone you love passes away. All other pain in life is ego based, and it may bruise you—even deeply—but your natural inclination is to heal over time.

That's not the case with soul-level pain. It can cause you to lock yourself inside your house and get ready for the next painful moment. Christmas? It's going to be painful, so you just avoid it. Your brother's birthday? You know it's going to be torture, and it *is*. I wanted my mom and I to power through that pain, so without even telling her, I booked some time for us at a health spa after Daniel's funeral. While we were there, we did small things that comforted us even if they didn't take away the ache we constantly felt. We walked outside in the sunshine. We took naps. We drank warm herbal tea and ate healthy food. We weren't looking for satisfaction; we were embracing the notion that micro actions of self-care are the tiny drops of happiness that can, one day, fill up a bucket of blessings. Our little moments of healthy living nourished us ever so slightly, clearing the path to allow us to see the work that still needed to be done in our lives in order to move forward toward happiness.

Let me be clear on one thing. After Daniel died, my mom and I were still fortunate to make a solid income from our family business. We weren't in debt then, and I'm so grateful we were able to spend money on our health and self-care. But you don't have to have *any* money to take care of yourself and, in this book, I won't ask you to. These twelve actions are free.

Why Start with Liquids till Lunch?

The first action in my program directs you to consume only liquids from the time you wake up until the time you eat lunch. In the next chapter, I'll get into the nitty-gritty of why "Liquids till Lunch" promotes better digestion, gives you more energy, and helps you lose weight—among other benefits. But, right now, I want to show you how this concept was a catalyst for my program and my company, MaryRuth Organics, and why it's a great starting place for this book.

Not long after my clients began doing Liquids till Lunch, many of them complained that taking vitamin capsules on an empty stomach made them feel queasy. That made total sense to me, so I figured: *Why not make a liquid multivitamin using wholesome ingredients and no sugar?* I searched and found a formulator and packager, then commissioned ninety bottles of a liquid raspberry multivitamin. (Ninety bottles isn't a lot, but we were still in debt.) I gave them out to my current batch of clients and crossed my fingers. Guess what? They *loved* it and reported that they'd had no nausea while doing Liquids till Lunch and taking the liquid multivitamin. Even better, they felt an instant boost of energy that prepared them for the day ahead.

I commissioned more bottles and decided to sell them on Amazon. When my liquid morning multivitamin went live online, it quickly got a good amount of five-star reviews. Because I was making a sugar-free liquid multivitamin, and similar products contained sugar, mine shot to the top of the Amazon algorithm and first page. Within one year, it sold well and helped so many people achieve better health and increased energy. MaryRuth Organics had been born!

This company freed my mom and me from $700,000 of debt within a few years, with zero outside funding and no investors. Seven years in, my family and over seventy employees are giving back by helping millions of Americans develop more energy, regain their health, heal themselves, and move forward in their lives. What I do gives me great contentment and satisfaction, and I'm moving forward every single day.

The beauty of Liquids till Lunch is that liquids are so much more absorbable than solids. They seep right into your cells, giving them all the good stuff that helps you function. They're also a refreshing start to the day: your first very simple and energetic move that provides the momentum for you to move forward.

That's why Liquids till Lunch is the perfect anchor for this book. The simple act of starting your day with only liquids is accessible to everyone, easily digestible, easy-to-follow, and free. Like the program I'll present to you in this book, you can seamlessly integrate it into your life without much effort or thought. As with every component of my program, it's completed within a short period of time, so you don't have to worry that you'll be toiling away or starving if you decide to follow the advice in this book. Liquids till Lunch was the start of one of the best things that ever happened in my life, and I hope, as the framework for my program, it can lead you down the road to a great quality of life, purpose, and happiness, too.

Move Forward Every Day

Claire was a busy working mother of two. She had a great job on Wall Street and enough money to hire a nanny and house-keeper and take cabs to and from work. A banker's salary can pay for most things, but what it can't buy is time, and Claire had none of that. Her early mornings were devoted to catching up on the previous night's emails and spending quality time with her children. Every second of the workday was devoted to clients, meetings, or phone calls. If she was lucky, she left work at 7 p.m., getting home just in time to sit down to the dinner she'd ordered on Postmates. Then she'd snuggle with her children, read them books, and tuck them in. After she caught up with her husband, watched a half-hour show, and checked email one last time, she was wiped out. In bed by 9:30 most nights, she slept like the dead, then got up at 5:30 a.m. the next day to do it all over again.

Claire loved her job and wouldn't entertain the thought of quitting, but the pace of her life was hurting her. Every single day, one after another, was the same sprint to the finish. She loved going to barre class before she had children, but now sacrificing even thirty minutes of sleep to exercise felt impossible. She never lost the baby weight, so the beautiful clothes she could afford made her feel frumpy. She was tired, unsatisfied, and torn in too many directions. She was a rock star on Wall Street and in the eyes of her family, so why didn't she feel like one? Claire needed physical, emotional, and spiritual healing, but she had absolutely no idea where to start. So she spilled her guts to a friend one Sunday afternoon at the playground.

"Take things one day at a time," her friend responded. "You can't expect to tackle your challenges all at once, so focus on making it through today."

Taking your life one day at a time is a cultural message we hear all the time, and while it helps people wake up, clock in, and make it till bedtime, in many ways living that way misses the point. You *must* think about the future. People like Claire already *are* living one day at a time, and that usually doesn't get them closer to happiness. In fact, it often makes them feel as if they're living the same suffocating day over and over again. In order to harness your full potential and operate to your highest-functioning degree, you need to *move forward every day*. You need to make gradual, incremental progress from one day to the next.

Language has power, so why use words that make you feel stagnant? Instead of numbering steps in my program, I describe "actions." Steps are a means for survival, but actions make you thrive. Action is something you can sink your teeth into. Action is sudden, fast, and decisive, like a director telling the camera to start rolling on a film or TV set. *Action!* Action propels you forward with purpose toward your goal, and gives you much more power than just living one day at a time.

Action Takes Consistent Hard Work

The minute you log on to social media, you're overwhelmed by *inspiration*. Everyone seems to have a simple yet visionary answer for everything, from what to eat in the morning to how to leave your abusive spouse. You want to make lots of money? It's easy! Stop caring about what anyone else thinks! Want to achieve true happiness? Learn to love yourself! Need to relax? Do yoga! I don't want to knock these perfectly logical, tried-and-true philosophies; I *totally* believe that you need to align yourself with what motivates you to get what you want. But these methods are confusing—especially to women, who so often feel pulled in opposite directions, and who suffer because they frequently put their own needs after everyone else's.

These pervasive cultural messages on social media are also incomplete. Nothing good in your life comes without working *consistently hard*. I'm not saying that you should wake up at 5 a.m. every day and kill yourself from sunup till sundown, but you have to strike a balance between understanding your purpose and creating a structure that allows you to get organized, feel motivated, and *act*. In no way, shape, or form am I dismissing self-care, either. Not only is taking care of yourself essential, that's what this book is about. But believing that relaxing, taking a deep breath, and warding off stress through a spiritual or physical practice alone is enough to propel you forward is a myth. The truth is that moving forward is a hard, multi-layered process that you'll have to work at consistently. Aligning yourself isn't the full story; you need to find your purpose and then put a lot of effort into it for the rest of your life.

Bear in mind the hard process you undertake to move forward might be gradual, but it's still profound. The power found in one action leads to another and, pretty soon, you're not just going through the motions of daily life but are, instead, taking true control of your actions. When Claire did Liquids till Lunch in the morning, she found she had the energy and desire to do push-ups and stretches before her children woke up. A bit of her zip returned, and she decided to start taking her children hiking on the weekend so she could bond with them and lose a little weight. Over time, she began to move forward in ways that were deeper and more consequential than simply surviving one day at a time, going from "thing to thing." The actions in this book empowered her to wrestle back control of her time and energy, and life stopped feeling like a daily slog. Claire turned her hard work toward her own self-care, which allowed her to stay focused on what her purpose was: to be the best working mom she could. Before long, she lived this mission daily, intentionally, and through every single one of her actions.

Structure Creates Freedom

Much of the work you need to do to move forward involves building a structure within your life. In this book, I'll distill that approach even further, giving you the tools to build a structure *within your day*. A daily structure might sound the tiniest bit restrictive to you. Whatever happened to flying by the seat of your pants? Trust me, on any given day you'll have the opportunity to make spur-of-the-moment decisions or go with your gut and decide to do one thing and not another.

I'm also not advocating a one-size-fits-all approach to your day. I firmly believe that everyone has their own method of operating, and the exact way I make green juice in the morning is not going to be yours. You know yourself and your needs best. The structure I'm talking about deals with very precise, fundamental ways you treat your body and mind within one twenty-four-hour period. If you know the night before that you'll be taking twelve actions that will provide crucial self-care to your routine tomorrow, I am confident it will provide comfort.

Comfort isn't the only benefit of structure, though. It gets even better—those who create the most structure have the *most freedom*. Whether you realize it or not, you most likely love order and dislike uncertainty because without a well-defined order within set parameters it's very easy to welcome in chaos. There are no rules, no direction, and no discipline. You don't know what your priorities are or where to start, and that's stressful. With structure, you are empowered to do whatever it is you need to do. You feel strong, capable, and energized.

My oldest son, Ethan, was born in May 2017. He was a beautiful baby with round, rosy cheeks and my husband's big brown eyes. He was also intelligent, funny, and incredibly kind. But at about eight months old, my mother's intuition kicked in and I finally admitted that something was clearly wrong. Ethan wouldn't crawl. He never tried to stand up. And he couldn't swallow solid foods like other babies. When Ethan was nine months old, I decided to speak with a physical therapist about my concerns.

"He'll be fine," she said, "Just wait and see. Some babies come to these things late."

So, I waited. I tiptoed into his room every morning, expecting to find him standing up. He never did. I fed him bananas during the day, expecting him not to spit them up. He usually did. Months passed, and nothing changed. I became pregnant again, gave birth to my second son, and when Ethan was fifteen months old and Elliot was just two weeks old, I decided that enough was enough.

My husband, David, and I took Ethan to a neurologist. We were called into a private room, where we put our son on the table. He sat like he always did: sweet and happy, but tired and inactive. The neurologist came in and was cordial, but he didn't say much. Instead, he gently pulled Ethan's arms, then pushed them back. He lifted his legs, then pulled and twisted them slightly. After a few minutes of this, he asked us to take Ethan off the table, then he sat down.

"I'm fairly certain your son has moderate hypotonia."

David and I didn't know what that meant. "Can you explain what that is?" I asked.

The doctor took a deep breath. "It means he has low muscle tone and restricted movement because of it. I can't tell you what he's facing will be easy, and it's going to require daily physical therapy and a lot of love to help him through it. But I need you to be prepared for the fact that there's a 30 percent chance he'll never walk. He may be bound to a wheelchair when he grows up."

I don't remember responding or leaving the room and neither does David. But when we walked back into the waiting room, we both remember bursting into tears.

Crying is a wonderful, cathartic release of emotions, but you can't do it all day. I still had to go to work, respond to my customers' emails, nurse my newborn, and deal with my raging postpartum hormones. I still had to carry my seventeen-month-old up and down the stairs every morning and night, pump breast milk, change two babies' diapers, and, if I was lucky, sleep more than three hours at a stretch.

Most importantly, I had to come up with a plan to get Ethan the help he needed. Over the next few days, I researched, I googled, and I chatted on message boards for parents of children with hypotonia. Eventually, I settled on an extensive plan that would push me to my limits, including three kinds of therapies—often multiple times a day, both in our house and at a clinic—and semiweekly visits with a feeding specialist. Some of these appointments would require me to drive half an hour each way, and many of them would go on indefinitely. A few of my friends asked, "Why don't you just wait and see if Ethan gets better before you do all this?" But I know the amount of development that happens before age three, so I hit the ground running.

You can deal with pain now or deal with pain later (one of my favorite mottoes), and I had no choice but to deal with Ethan's struggles now. *My* pain was a different story, though. I knew that if I shoved the depressing realization that I had a special-needs son under the rug, I might paralyze myself with indecision and denial. If I couldn't move forward, neither would my son.

I decided to implement the twelve actions into my life even more seriously to create greater structure, routine, and organization. I felt such gratitude for the time and self-care they provided, and they gave me ownership over something during a time that felt immensely chaotic and overwhelming. Once again, the twelve actions gave my life a routine and returned my power—the power I needed to help my son. They put me in a positive place, and that gave me confidence.

The twelve actions also gave me *freedom*. That freedom wasn't about having all the time in the world—trust me, I had none of that. It was a feeling, a sensation of lightness, that anything was possible. I had a daily routine to carry out, I could see the big picture, and I could visualize how to tackle it. And I knew that if anything bad happened, like Ethan's treatment going south or his pediatrician delivering bad news, I was organized and energetic enough to deal with it.

I believe the twelve actions are a huge reason Ethan can walk today.

Healing Through Repetition

As you follow my program, you'll be doing the same things day after day. The saying goes that practice makes perfect, and never is that truer than with healing. The more you act deliberately in the interest of self-care, the more energy you develop. With more energy comes greater momentum. Pushing forward, you can dislodge yourself from the obstacles that hinder you and work toward whatever goal or goals you have in mind.

Stanford behavioral scientist B. J. Fogg created a breakthrough program called "Tiny Habits," which he describes in detail in the *New York Times* bestselling book of the same name. Dr. Fogg writes that implementing tiny, helpful behaviors into your routine, then repeating them daily, will allow you to develop healthy habits. The more healthy habits you allow to take root in your life, the richer and more productive you will be. My program *gives* you a road map to the tiny habits that you can make part of your life, so you won't be left scratching your head, unable to figure out where to begin. You can start with any one of the twelve actions that sound interesting to you.

In 2020, I saw how healing through repetition worked in my little corner of the world. I decided to write this book in February, just a few weeks before COVID-19 slammed into the United States like a head-on collision. I live in Los Angeles, and when the governor ordered everyone in California to stay home, I had to run my company and write this book while I was locked inside with my husband and our two toddlers. I'd also just found out I was pregnant with twins, and I was throwing up at least four times a day (which went on for *five months*). The joy I felt at having my family and this book in my life was huge, but the pain I suffered as I watched businesses collapse, friends get sick, and hospitals fill up was over the top. I was literally trapped inside my house and figuratively inside my fear over what was happening to the world. Not to mention, I was a prisoner of my miserable, pregnant body and bone-crushing nausea.

I know millions of you out there felt the same—and worse—and I'm deeply empathetic to that. Few of us knew how bad things would get or how long they'd stay that way, and almost all of us felt confused, angry, and hopeless. This book is not about me, politics, society, or the virus, so it won't be my diary of the pandemic. Yes, every day felt like a crisis in the first few weeks, and, in crisis, there can be great change. However, profound realizations unfold over time, and I don't want my overall thoughts about this global tragedy to be impulsive, so I will pause and let my reflections simmer, providing no conclusions yet.

What I will say about the COVID-19 pandemic is something I witnessed right at the beginning of quarantine. I noticed that, day after day, many of us decided to protect ourselves, boost our immune systems, radiate positive energy, and study up on the science and data that would assure us that, yes, we could handle this. Self-care became an essential daily activity, so millions of us went for solitary walks on the beach, sat in the sun, or practiced yoga online. We hugged our children more. We framed pictures and cleaned closets. We cooked nourishing meals. We remembered how nice it is to call our friends and family.

Remember those good feelings, because I want you to find them here, in this book. It is meant to be comforting when you need to feel good and get your life back in control. By giving you easy, accessible actions and tools for self-care, it will help you generate a positive energy that's both deeply personal and universal. It won't magically solve all your problems, but it will give you the means to pause, reflect, and be a little kinder to yourself. Most of all, it will grant you the resources to move forward, whatever path you choose.

Liquids till Lunch

Eat three small meals a day, at the anchor times of noon, 3 p.m., and 7 p.m. Make sure to hit all three anchor times!

When I met Naomi, she was a stay-at-home mom who'd left her marketing job a few months after the birth of her twin girls, who were now one. She and her husband had worked hard and saved money, so she knew that unless something unexpected or bad happened, they wouldn't feel any financial stress for at least a few years. Naomi hired a sitter a few days a week so she was able to go to the gym, meet friends for lunch, and do her grocery shopping without her children along.

Even though Naomi had a strong marriage, lots of friends, and help at home, she was depressed. She loved being there for her girls and felt that she was always meant to be a stay-at-home mom—at least before they went to preschool—but she was empty inside. She desperately missed getting out of the house and going to the office every day, where the millennials she'd worked with talked about the TV shows they were binge watching rather than nap schedules and teething. She hated rushing home from the gym, worried she might be late for her sitter. A year ago, her free time had been her own, but now it seemed to be everyone else's. She also missed feeling like her brain was on fire with deadlines and data, and she yearned for the satisfaction of pushing "send" on a presentation she'd worked on for weeks. When she woke up at 6 a.m. to the sound of two little voices she loved with all her heart, she was foggy and resentful, and it wasn't only because of the three glasses of wine she'd had the night before to unwind. When she poured her second cup of coffee and nibbled on her daughter's leftover waffle, praying it would settle her hangover, she felt exhausted. It was only 7 a.m. Was this what the rest of her life was going to be like?

I'm not a licensed mental health professional, so I immediately told Naomi that I wouldn't be able to diagnose any emotional problems she might be having, though it was clear to me she was anxious and depressed. While I suggested that having three glasses of wine at night might be disrupting her sleep pattern (it was; more on that in action seven), I didn't feel I knew her well enough to tell her she might have a drinking problem. Nor was it my place. Instead, I pulled a marker out of my desk drawer, placed a piece of paper in front of Naomi, and drew a circle.

"We're dividing your day into one-hour chunks," I said, making lines for each hour. "It seems like morning is a tough time for you, so I'm going to block it off and give it some structure. If I can streamline the most difficult hours of the day for you *and* show you how you can easily and quickly nourish yourself on a cellular level, I can promise you're going to feel more alive. With more energy, you're going to be able to move forward every single day."

Then I introduced her to the first action in my program: Liquids till Lunch.

The Energetic Foundation of Liquids till Lunch

Following Liquids till Lunch is simple. After you wake up in the morning, you can drink water, coffee, green juice, vegetable broth, milk, or tea until lunchtime. If you take vitamins in the morning, try liquid vitamins rather than pills, because they won't cause nausea. Avoid sugary beverages and fruit juice because they'll spike your blood sugar and lead to hunger (more on that later in this chapter), but drink anything else you want, as much as you want. Liquids fill you up and help stop food cravings.

The first benefit of following Liquids till Lunch is that you'll have more energy. This comes as a shock to most people, and they worry: *Isn't breakfast the most important meal of the day? What's going to give me energy if I don't have anything in my stomach?* The truth is that your body already has the energy it needs stored away in your liver and in your fat cells. When you don't eat, your levels of insulin—a hormone produced by the pancreas that signals it's time to metabolize food—fall. Your digestive system then realizes there's nothing to burn, and it turns to your liver for energy. The liver metabolizes a chain of stored sugars called *glycogen*, converts the glycogen into glucose, and releases the glucose into your bloodstream. This raises your blood-sugar levels, giving your body an instant boost of energy. If your liver doesn't have enough glycogen, your body turns its attention to fat cells. Fat takes longer than food or glycogen to metabolize, but it's a great and ready source of energy. Better yet, breaking it down is what causes you to lose cellulite on your thighs and belly.

See? You have plenty of energy reserves. When you skip a meal, there's no chance you're going to wither away or starve to death.

Okay, you're thinking. *All this is great, but will I feel like I have more energy?* Yes. At the same time your body is burning glycogen or fat in the absence of food, the body ramps up its level of counterregulatory hormones, including noradrenaline, growth hormone, and cortisol. These are the "stress hormones" produced by the adrenal glands. Together they increase responsiveness, speed up your heart rate, raise your blood pressure, and activate your body's fight-or-flight response. With all those extra hormones rushing through your system, does that mean you're going to be a nervous wreck, have tense muscles, and feel like your heart might leap out of your chest? I've been following Liquids till Lunch for over ten years, and that's never happened. Every one of the clients I've taught this method to have said the same; they aren't on edge or panicky. Their energy is deep yet expansive in a way it's never been before. The more Liquids till Lunch becomes a part of their routine, the more they develop what I call "Eye of the Tiger."

Eye of the Tiger

Imagine you're a tiger on the hunt. There's no food in your belly, but you're sharp, laser-focused, and ready for action. You're ready to rise up and go the distance in order to survive. Driven by an intense competitive edge, you aren't afraid of a challenge. You have the energy to do almost anything, so you're like a guided missile, powering toward your destination.

That's Eye of the Tiger. It's focused, high-level function and, as the theme song from *Rocky* says, the thrill of the fight.

The reason you gain the Eye of the Tiger when you practice Liquids till Lunch is because, as studies show, intermittent fasting—which I define as skipping at least one meal you'd normally eat on a regular basis—doesn't affect your mind. Two recent studies that measured brain function after both a twenty-four-hour fast and a two-day fast revealed that reaction time, memory, mood, and function were not impaired during either period without food.

Evolution points to the benefits of fasting, too. Our ancestors didn't have food delivery services or grocery stores. They were hunter/gatherers, and sometimes their crops didn't grow, or the prey went in the other direction. These ancient people went long periods without eating, yet they adapted and survived. To do this, their bodies conserved energy by shrinking all their organs except for two. One was the testicles because they were needed for reproduction. The other was the brain. Our ancestors had to stay sharp to find food, so they developed Eye of the Tiger.

The Gift of Time

Time is the great equalizer. You could be the richest, most successful person in America, or you could be working two jobs while raising a family. For each person, there are only twenty-four hours in a day and 365 days in a year.

If you want to move forward or out of a situation that's keeping you stagnant, or if you dream of taking your life to the next level, those hours and days are precious. If you're a new graduate fresh out of college, you need optimism and a competitive edge to beat out the other thousand-something candidates who are applying for the same entry-level job as you. If you're a plumber in a town with five other plumbers who have better ratings on Google and Yelp than you do, you need great ideas and a big vision to make yourself stand out. You have to get up in the morning fresh as a daisy and ready to conquer the world, and then you need to hit the ground running. If you don't, chances are you'll be left behind.

Liquids till Lunch gives you time you thought you didn't have. It reminds me of a former client who bought a membership to a bike-sharing service so that he could bike to the subway rather than walk. He saved five minutes each way, but those ten extra minutes totaled fifty by the end of the week. When my client did the math and realized what he'd gained, he decided to fit in an extra workout one morning a week. It was like time had appeared out of thin air.

The primary caregivers within families love these extra minutes more than anyone. If you're Naomi, you don't have to stop and scarf down a hangover-helper breakfast while you're rushing off to your children's playgroup. Most parents don't just yearn for a few extra minutes in the day; often they literally search for reasons not to think about themselves and their needs so they can turn their attention to their children, the dishes, or packing school lunches. I think putting self-care last is a terrible idea, but the truth is it's what a lot of moms and dads do. Luckily—and

> ## MOVE FORWARD EVERY DAY
>
> Green juice is a super healthy and delicious way to start your morning. Just always be sure to drink it on an empty stomach at least half an hour before a meal so that your digestive system can rapidly absorb all its nutrients. If you drink green juice with food in your belly, your cells won't get all those vitamins and minerals as easily.

paradoxically—conserving time and energy through Liquids till Lunch gives these same people space to focus on their macro needs, their larger purpose, and how they can break down the obstacles that stand in their way.

The Benefits of Better Digestion

I love to use visualization to help people change their habits and behavior, and this exercise is one of my favorites:

Imagine you're standing in a large room with no furniture. There's so much space you can dance and do cartwheels, and you feel free and light as air. Now, turn your attention to the dump truck that's backing up toward the room. The glass doors of the room swing open, and as the back of the truck tilts down, 365 breakfasts spill out. Bowls of cereal, plates of eggs, home fries, and muffins tumble on top of each other.

There's so much food you could probably feed a small army, but this massive spread is what you've fed yourself for a year.

Sit and stare at that mountain of junk. How do you feel? Tired, bloated, or constipated? Don't worry. This is just pretend, and it'll be over soon. Now, imagine all that food disappearing. Over the course of a year, that's food that doesn't have to go in your mouth, down your esophagus, into your stomach and small intestine, through your large intestine, and out your body. For a few hours a day, your digestive system gets a much-needed rest, allowing your body to devote energy to other essential functions.

Your digestive system finally has a chance to relax and repair on a cellular level with Liquids till Lunch because, when there's not food in your body, it can turn its attention to other things. Your enzymes can tackle digestive ailments, from simple imbalances or sensitivities (due to eating too much or the wrong types of foods) to more serious conditions like colitis or inflammatory bowel disease. Rather than metabolizing food, your enzymes can work on breaking down and filtering out toxins that circulate in your system.

Finally, your gut is full of millions of microorganisms that aid in digestion, and fasting has been shown to help keep a healthy balance among all of them. A 2016 study by the Proceedings of the National Academy of Sciences demonstrated that, in fruit flies—who have metabolism-related genes that are similar to humans—fasting turns on a molecular pathway in the brain that activates an anti-inflammatory response in your gut. This brain–belly reaction protects your healthy digestive bacteria and reduces your risk for gastrointestinal diseases.

The benefits of improved gut health and digestion are cumulative. Better balanced intestinal flora one day leads to a reduced risk of disease the next. A well-functioning gastrointestinal tract that's had a few hours to rest results in higher energy and more efficient body systems. Greater efficiency and higher levels of energy then lead to better brain function, improved sleep, fewer illnesses, and more. If you're sleeping, thinking, and feeling better, you get closer and closer to becoming your personal best. Day after day and year after year, you grow a little stronger, you don't look or feel as old, and you have more pep in your step. All this started because you stopped eating solid foods in the morning.

Everything in my program is about the cumulative effects of good health, starting at the cellular level. When you don't put food in your belly in the morning, you gradually build up your body and mind. That one bowl of cereal doesn't become 365 by the end of the year. The micro step of skipping breakfast and replacing it with liquids leads to the macro, manifesting a beautiful tool that gives you greater energy and a generous amount of brand-new time. Who doesn't want that?

Liquids till Lunch Makes You Look Good

Probably the most well-publicized benefit of intermittent fasting is weight loss. There's a common misperception that the pounds will start to fly off because not eating breakfast means you're consuming fewer calories during the day. Fewer calories into your digestive system mean less energy to store away as fat. A reduction in fat storage means weight loss, right?

Not quite. Fat burning is a hormonal response regulated by insulin. It's not about how many calories you take in versus how many you burn, but rather how balanced your blood-sugar levels are.

Let me give you an example to illustrate this. Craig was a thirty-nine-year-old client of mine who'd carried about thirty extra pounds since his late twenties. He'd just broken up with his long-term girlfriend, and even though part of him was relieved the relationship was over, a bigger part of him felt lonely and depressed. He didn't want to dip mentally lower before he turned forty, so he decided that losing weight would boost his self-esteem. He joined a gym and invested money in a calorie-restricted diet program. Craig hit the treadmill religiously every day after work, making sure he burned at least 500 calories. He meticulously counted calories, trying as hard as possible not to exceed 2,500. He'd read that 2,000 calories a day was the magic number that would allow him to lose a pound a week, so time on the treadmill would bring him down to that. He ate three meals a day with two snacks in between, and while he didn't go overboard on carbs, he didn't restrict them, either. Cereal for breakfast was fine, and so was a whole-grain granola bar for his midmorning snack. As long as Craig stayed under his calorie limit, he thought he could have beer, pasta, and even the occasional dessert.

Unfortunately, Craig didn't lose any weight, and his self-esteem was lower than it had been in years. The problem was that Craig's diet was keeping his blood sugar high all day long. Carbs are easily metabolized sugars, and he ate them at every meal, five times a day. Insulin rushed into his system in response to them, and his blood sugar spiked. We'll talk more in action five about the healthy, whole foods you should be eating to feel your best, but know this for now: When you eat less often—such as when you skip breakfast—your insulin levels drop. This tells your body that there's no food available to metabolize. As I said before, your body then has to burn the energy it has stored as glycogen or, if that's gone, fat. Guess what fat burning leads to? Weight loss. Fasting also increases your metabolism, which means you burn energy more efficiently. Your body hums along like a well-oiled machine, using the available energy stores efficiently rather than getting bogged down sifting through a pile of food stacked up in your belly. Like you, it has Eye of the Tiger, focused on making the most of its available time and working to the highest-functioning degree.

Weight loss doesn't necessarily happen right away, but it will happen over time. As soon as a few weeks after making Liquids till Lunch part of your life, you may notice subtle shifts in weight. Your jeans might fit better. Your face might look less full, and you may experience less gas pressure.

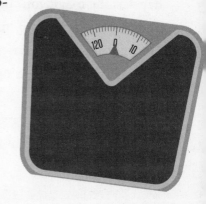

Everyone's body is different, so I can't promise that you'll lose two pounds or twenty, but *something* will happen to you. You might feel lighter, stronger, or less tense. Someone on Instagram told me that she'd finally done a handstand in her yoga class after months of trying and failing. Craig ended up losing fifteen pounds in three months, and he said he felt confident and in control in a way he hadn't in years.

Control is the key word here. By carrying out one small action every day, you gradually—but cumulatively—begin to take control of a situation you thought was out of your grasp. Liquids till Lunch is a micro action that can lead to macro change, and that's not just about your waistline. Losing a few pounds will give you energy. Better energy leads to a competitive edge. And a competitive edge may help you transform whatever situation is preventing you from moving forward.

Going Outside Your Comfort Zone

I completely get the fact that Liquids till Lunch might be intimidating to some of you. Breakfast can be a cherished ritual you've had since childhood. Think of lazy Sunday mornings when you woke up to the smell of frying eggs at your grandma's house, or the bowl of cereal your mom would have ready for you and your brother before you dashed out to the school bus. Won't letting go of these routines make you unhappy? You might be surprised that it doesn't feel like a big deal, or you may realize that you can always eat breakfast foods for lunch or dinner. Skipping breakfast may also feel unnatural. After twelve or so hours without any food, isn't your body desperate for food, and won't you be starving if you don't eat?

This part of learning to move forward every day involves going outside your comfort zone. Pushing boundaries or taking risks may be hard work, and it may not always feel good, but it's necessary. I never would have experienced the profound satisfaction I have with my company if I'd stayed in my very stable real estate job that brought in a great paycheck but only made me feel so-so. Someone who goes running after years of no exercise is definitely going to feel their muscles burn and their heart race. This discomfort signals growth. Plus, putting yourself in a potentially scary, uncomfortable situation gives you the knowledge, skills, and tools to overcome your fears—or even just live with them. Fears stand in the way of your ability to function at the highest-possible degree, but taking one micro step to move past them will help you grow by leaps and bounds.

Pretty quickly, Liquids till Lunch will also get easier for you. Your body will become stronger and more efficient, and your cravings will go down. That occasional hunger may be unpleasant, but there is absolutely no reason to fear Liquids till Lunch; mild hunger pangs are your body's signal that it's burning stored glycogen or fat. It's telling you you're doing something good for yourself healthwise, and you're training yourself to test your limits and overcome the discomfort that's inevitable in life.

Hunger pangs are also easy to deal with. First, you should drink more liquids because often what people assume to be hunger is actually thirst. Liquids fill your belly up and activate your stomach's stretch receptors, which signal to your brain that you're full, even if you aren't. Coffee or tea is especially helpful because caffeine suppresses your appetite for a short period of time.

You can also chew sugar-free gum, because it satisfies your sweet tooth and tricks your brain into thinking you're eating something. Try not to chew too much (meaning about a pack a day), because most sugar-free gum contains chemical ingredients in the form of sweeteners, flavorings, and preservatives. There are nontoxic gums available, though, with ingredients like natural gum base and stevia, and they taste great. Always chew gum with your mouth closed, because you swallow air when you chew with an open mouth, and air in your belly creates uncomfortable gas pressure.

Next, try exercising first thing in the morning. Research shows that people who exercise regularly tend to experience less hunger than those who don't.

Finally, work at getting a better night's sleep. If you sleep at least seven hours a night, I promise you'll have fewer cravings in the morning.

If nothing but food heals your hunger before noon, eating a piece of fruit is absolutely acceptable!

The Pushback Theory

You may have days you can't stand the idea of skipping breakfast and that's fine. Or you might wake up, roll out of bed, feel great . . . and then feel so famished by 10 a.m. that you have to eat. That's also okay! You don't need to suffer to make change, and you don't have to follow Liquids till Lunch every single day to experience its benefits. Just work at it as best you can, and it will become part of your routine at the time that's best for you.

The Pushback Theory promotes the idea that you should push back your lunchtime as much as possible, but only as far as you're comfortable. The more you work at Liquids till Lunch, the stronger you'll become, but don't torture yourself. Just be patient and realize that a great deal of power lies in taking one positive action. The most important part of moving forward is productivity, and if you can make it one or two extra hours without eating, that's one or two hours of extra time and energy.

Eating your breakfast bowl at 8:00 a.m. rather than 7:00 a.m. is a massive step for someone who's stuck in a bad situation. You need to meet yourself where you are and *own* that accomplishment. That one extra hour may turn to two the following day,

MOVE FORWARD EVERY DAY

If you're about to get on an airplane, try to eat about half an hour before you board. If you absolutely must eat on a plane, do it only once. Food doesn't digest well at a high altitude, so you can develop digestive problems, such as bloating or constipation.

then three after that. After slipping for a day because you didn't get enough sleep the night before and are hungry, you might bounce right back and make it till 11 a.m. by the end of the week. Your micro steps will add up to macro actions as long as you keep at it, moving forward toward your goals.

Action Through Anchor Times

"Structure creates freedom." Remember that from the introduction? I want you to make that your motto during the times you eat. Your macro goal is to have the kind of peak energy that will power you through the day, giving you focus and the freedom to do what your heart desires. I promise you, you'll have that if you schedule your meals and snack times precisely following what I call *anchor times*. Scientists, doctors, and nutritionists disagree on what times work best for your digestive and adrenal systems, so I've based my program on how people who are working 9-to-5 jobs, picking up their children from school, or going to lunch meetings schedule their time.

- **FIRST LUNCH:** Eat a reasonably sized meal around 12 or 1 p.m. This meal should make you feel full but not over-stuffed. You don't have to *finish* your food within that time, but aim to start eating then.

- **SECOND LUNCH:** You should eat a small meal or healthy snack around 3 or 4 p.m. If you went to a restaurant for first lunch, you can eat something you brought back to work in a to-go bag. You can also eat the sandwich you didn't finish at first lunch. Or pick up something new!

- **DINNER:** This is a reasonably sized meal you consume around 7 or 8 p.m. Your commute is over, you're home from work, it's time to eat!

If you work the night shift or have irregular hours, never fear. Just adjust your anchor times into three- to four-hour increments based on when you plan to eat.

Eating only at anchor times may be a bit of an adjustment for a lot of people, but that's because of how we've been conditioned as a society to think about food. Satchin Panda, a biologist at the Salk Institute in La Jolla, California, and author of the book *The Circadian Code* writes that most Americans eat their meals over the course of fifteen hours. They wake up around 7 a.m. and don't stop eating till they turn the TV off at 10 p.m. and put on their PJs. I'm not a research biologist, but I'm guessing that fifteen hours of food consists of three meals and about four to five snacks, right? Just know that this pattern of eating is not ideal for your digestive tract, so I urge you to avoid the temptation to graze or eat outside of your set anchor times.

Your body has a network of internal clocks that tell your cells when to regulate internal functions such as sleep cycles, the release of hormones, blood pressure, mood stabilization, and more. Collectively, this system is known as your body's circadian rhythm.

The cells within our digestive system have internal clocks that prepare them for the arrival of food. Your esophagus, stomach, intestines, liver, pancreas, and more have hard work to do, from breaking down the food to metabolizing it to storing it as fat or glycogen, and they have to be ready. Digestion is an intricate dance among your various tissues, organs, and cells, and if they're not in harmony, problems can develop. You might get gas or bloating in the short term, or, over time, you might develop type 2 diabetes or metabolic syndrome.

Your biochemistry operates better or worse depending on the time of day and when the digestive system has had time to rest

MOVE FORWARD EVERY DAY

Want to be even stronger and peppier in the morning? Start your day with a freezing cold shower followed by Liquids till Lunch. The icy cold water against your body wakes you up (obviously), but it also gives you a rush of adrenaline and norepinephrine, which increase energy and focus. Cold water improves blood circulation, which reduces muscle soreness, and constricts your blood vessels, which improves your immune system. Finally, it pushes you way past your comfort zone, testing your limits and uncovering the tough stuff you need to move forward.

and digest at regular intervals. If your cells' internal clocks are off, though, everything goes crazy in your gut. Think about how you feel after a long flight. Your body is tired and your brain is foggy from jet lag, but the problems don't stop there. The digestive system regulates at a different rate than your tissues, so a massive time change throws off your body's internal balance. With jet lag, you may become constipated, feel bloated, or suffer from indigestion, signaling that your digestive system isn't operating at its highest-functioning degree.

Why the particular periods of time I've chosen, though? Because after you've eaten your first meal of the day, your energy dips as digestion steals it from the rest of your body. If you power up with a small meal at 3 or 4 p.m., you'll be giving yourself an energy boost just when other people are winding down, thinking about dinnertime. If you then eat at 7 or 8, your energy will dip around 10 or 11, right when it's time for bed.

Anchor-time eating is about giving your body the control and certainty it needs. With certainty comes efficiency, and with efficiency comes more energy. The same holds true for Liquids till Lunch. You might have so much energy in the morning that your outlook will improve in subtle ways that soon become profound. When Naomi stopped picking at her children's food and drinking green juice instead, she felt so revitalized that she stopped snapping at her girls in the morning. Emboldened by her better attitude, she began to drink less at night. Within a few weeks, she'd lost three pounds and, suddenly, she felt like herself again.

2.

Chew Your Food
Until It Becomes Liquid

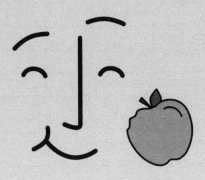

Jessica was an incredibly sweet, hardworking forty-year-old single woman who had the kind of positive attitude that could get her through anything. So, when she decided she was sick of living in the run-down rental apartment she'd shared with the boyfriend she'd broken up with the year before, the idea of looking for her own condo thrilled her. She'd never owned anything as major as a car or apartment before, and her own home—which she could paint all the colors that made her happy and renovate just to her style—felt like a beautiful fresh start. Her friends promised they'd go to open houses with her, and her mom recommended a broker. But when Jessica added up closing costs, the monthly mortgage, condo fees, and property taxes, she was shocked. Jessica made good money as a magazine editor and had a lot saved up, but it wasn't enough for a down payment and hiring a real estate lawyer, while still putting food on the table. It was time for a *huge* raise.

Jessica was full of courage about finding her dream home, but she wasn't always that way at the office. She worked long hours and was wonderful at her job, but she'd always just assumed that her company compensated her at the level she deserved. Or . . . did it? The truth was that Jessica had never asked around, done any research, or pushed the issue. She'd been happy at the magazine for almost twenty years, and she trusted her bosses because they were kind and supportive. Plus, she hadn't really needed the extra money. Now she did, and she asked herself if it was possible that her inadequate salary was a problem *she'd* created.

"I can't stick my neck out there and ask for a big raise, MaryRuth," she told me one day. "I'm the nice girl at the office, not the pushy one."

Jessica was so open that we talked about everything in our sessions. She'd come to me to tackle her frequent exhaustion and irritable bowel syndrome, so I decided that those issues were what we were going to focus on first. I also understood that by working through her health problems, Jessica would soon be able to turn her attention to her deep-seated fear of advocating for herself. She'd clear out internal obstacles, and that would allow her to tackle her external ones. Jessica began following my program, and within a month, she was less tired, and her digestive problems improved. As she became less worried about her health and got out of bed without pushing snooze five times, she felt like a cloud had been lifted from her. Her mind sharpened, and her confidence went up. After six weeks, she walked like a pro into her boss's office and made a strong case for a raise. Guess what? She got it!

It turns out she didn't have to change her external environment by working longer hours or looking for a new job; she just needed to shine a spotlight on her *herself.* She resolved the physical issues that were impacting her daily life and was able to access her internal strength and clarity of mind. By training her body to function at a higher, more efficient, and more energetic level, she unlocked the courage to ask for what she deserved.

When I became a certified health educator, I realized that every single person who came to see me came not because the outside world was holding them back, but because their own bodies and minds were. Without exception, my clients needed help with at least one of three things: losing weight, gaining more energy, or overcoming a health challenge. Maybe these people also felt stuck because of a death or job loss, or maybe they wanted a good life situation to become even better, but, when I dug a little deeper, I discovered that their internal issues were the true roadblocks to happiness. Their bodies felt out of control, and that loss of self-mastery affected every decision they made and every situation they dove into (or didn't dive into). When my clients entered with skin rashes, autoimmune diseases, joint pain, excess weight, chronic fatigue, or more, those health problems robbed them of their power and prevented them from moving forward. I knew they had to create balance on the inside to maintain balance on the outside, so I challenged them with the hardest action in my entire program. When I start to talk about it, you're probably going to laugh and think, *No way! That sounds so easy!* It's not. Believe me, this second action is *tough*.

The Power of Chewing Your Food Until It Becomes Liquid

Chewing your food until it's liquid holds tons of power. In fact, it can completely boost your energy level by jump-starting your digestive process.

Most people believe that digestion begins when the food you've eaten hits your stomach. This is false. Digestion starts when you bite into a piece of food and the glands on the inside of your mouth, under your tongue, and beneath your jawbone secrete saliva. When that saliva lubricates the food in your mouth, and your teeth begin to rip, grind, mash, and crush it, the process known as *mastication* has begun.

Mastication isn't the only thing that happens before you swallow. On a microscopic level, the salivary enzymes amylase and lipase start to break down the fats and carbohydrates in the food you're eating, helping your body absorb them more easily. When you feel ready to swallow, your tongue then moves the partially or fully liquified food bits to the back of your mouth and into your esophagus. This 10-inch-long organ also has salivary glands, and the saliva produced by these lubricate the food even more as it moves down toward the stomach in a series of muscular contractions called *peristalsis*.

Boom! Your food finally lands in your stomach. It's going to break down even more there, right? Sort of, but not like you think. The stomach doesn't have teeth, so no chopping or grinding happens in it. Strong muscles line the inside of the stomach, but they don't mash, they just churn and mix food around so that the volume squeezed into your small intestine is liquified and isn't too big. Acids and enzymes are what break down nutrients, but they only act on what they can touch, which is the surface of food particles. They don't actually penetrate or dig into food.

When what you've eaten and swallowed finally exits your stomach and enters the small intestine, it's met by enzymes from the pancreas and bile from the liver. These enzymes mix with the now-liquified food and break down its nutrients even further. Your food travels about 10 to 15 inches through the duodenum, or top part of the small intestine, then reaches the lower parts, the jejunum and the ileum, where the process of absorption begins.

All along the route of the small intestine, waste products are filtered out so your body can eliminate them. Anything that's not absorbable—including fiber, which gives bulk to food and helps create solid stools—passes into your large intestine. This rope-like organ pushes waste products toward your colon and rectum, where your body eliminates it.

The entire digestive process—from the moment food enters your mouth to the minute it leaves your body—takes approximately forty-two to forty-four hours and requires about 10 percent of the caloric energy you take in. The rest of your energy goes to muscular function, brain activity, heart rate, cellular repair, and every other bodily function required to live and breathe on this planet. So, my question is: Don't you want to save some of that precious energy for the things that *really* matter, like playing with your children, falling madly in love, getting your dream job, and moving forward toward your real purpose? Every speck of energy in your body matters, so why waste it in your stomach? The muscles in your jaw are some of the strongest and most efficient in your body, so give the work to them.

The fact is, when you swallow chunks of food rather than liquid, you absorb fewer nutrients, and that means less energy to go around. Your taste buds signal to your salivary glands how much saliva they need to secrete, and if you swallow too fast, you bypass the mixing of food and saliva. This prevents the digestion of many essential starches and sugars. These nutrients should have been broken down in the mouth, but instead they passed into the stomach, where it's harder to metabolize them. If you'd given your teeth the job they were born to do, they could have seamlessly turned that food into liquid, which would have allowed your body to absorb the nutrients it needs to function and thrive.

When we chew our food into tiny particles or liquid, we also create a greater surface area on every morsel that enters our digestive tract. Since digestive enzymes only work on the surface, creating more surface area means you can metabolize the entire meal rather than just parts of it. More food metabolized means more energy-boosting essential vitamins and minerals entering your system. You get all the benefits of enjoying a delicious meal from the taste to the multitude of nutrients!

Finally, when you swallow chunks of food rather than liquifying them in your mouth, you steal energy from one part of your body and give it to your relatively inefficient stomach. It takes more energy for the stomach to break down food than it does your mouth, so blood rushes to your belly from other parts of your body, delivering cellular energy that could have gone to other essential functions. Ever wonder why you feel tired after inhaling a huge meal? It's because your brain has literally been deprived of energy, and your body shuts down, desperate to conserve what little it has left.

Chewing for Weight Loss

John was a successful lawyer at a large New York City nonprofit. Years before, he'd worked at a corporate law firm making twice what he made at the nonprofit, but he'd never really felt comfortable there. The work itself was interesting, but his colleagues were *completely* obsessed with their jobs, and John craved a healthy work/life balance.

John's dissatisfaction came to a head during the Northeast blackout in August 2003. When the lights blinked off just before 5 p.m. and everyone left to go home, John walked back to his apartment, which was about a mile away. He woke up the next morning, noticed there was still no power, and expected that he wouldn't have to go into work. But when he checked his voice mail, it turns out that his bosses expected him at the office right on time, just as always. He put on a suit, hailed a cab, got to the office, and climbed up ten flights of stairs because the elevator wasn't operating. It was sweltering, and by the time he reached the top, his shirt was soaked with sweat. When he opened the door to his office, he couldn't believe what he saw: the air conditioning was off, the blinds and windows were up so light and air would come in, and his colleagues were sitting at their desks, pouring over files and writing briefs by hand.

MOVE FORWARD EVERY DAY

Because green juices and smoothies are both good for you, I think adding them to your diet during Liquids till Lunch is a great idea. But bear in mind they're not the same. The juicing process extracts fiber, so green juice contains little to none of it. The lack of fiber, however, makes all the nutrients packed in one glass more easily digestible, absorbable, and bioavailable to your cells. If you do drink green juice, drink it on an empty stomach so that your body takes in these nutrients more easily and so you don't get gas and bloating.

Smoothies are made of crushed fruits and vegetables that still contain all their natural fiber. Fiber is bulky and undigestible, but it's essential to the digestive process because it absorbs water, which helps stools pass through the large intestine more easily.

Really? John thought. *It's over 100 degrees in here. This is unsafe. Why am I expected to be at my desk?*

John stayed the day and gave his two-week notice the following morning. Within a month, he had a new job at a nonprofit—which hadn't expected their employees to come in during the blackout—and he was happier and more in balance then he'd ever been.

With extra time on his hands, John started jogging. Soon, he was entering himself in half marathons, then marathons. He ran the New York City Marathon every year starting at age thirty, and he improved his finishing time every year.

Just after John turned forty, he was walking down the street while texting, tripped, and broke his ankle. While he was recovering, he started to pack on weight. John couldn't run, of course, but he was also filling himself up with snacks and bigger meals than he used to eat. He ate out of boredom and because he was out of sorts without the structure provided by his daily jogs. Soon, his face looked puffy, his once-muscular arms got flabby, and he had trouble recognizing himself.

When John finally recovered, he decided to start running again, but struggled with his loss of muscle and the extra fifteen pounds he'd packed on. He began seeing me in the hopes of regaining his competitive edge, but when we talked about his interests, his work, and his history, I realized competition wasn't what he was looking for.

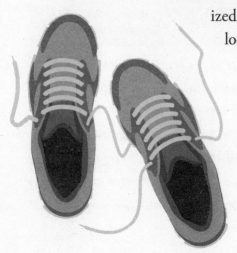

It was self-mastery.

"I know I'm a runner," John said, "but crossing the finish line before everyone else isn't what gets me out there. I hated the rat race and pressure to become partner at my old firm. It was just not me!"

When I talked to John, I was reminded of a quote I love from Lewis Howes, a former professional football player and the *New York Times* bestselling author of *The School of Greatness*. Lewis writes, "Your competition isn't other people. Your competition is your procrastination. Your ego. The unhealthy food that you're consuming, the knowledge you neglect. The negative behavior you're nurturing and your lack of creativity. Compete against that."

I knew that the motivation John would need to lose weight and lace up his running shoes again wouldn't come from a medal around his neck. He'd get it when, like Jessica, he looked inside and challenged himself to regain the power he had over his own body.

"You're going to love this, John," I said, "because the way you're going to lose this weight is like running a race during every meal. It's a competition with yourself that's going to take concentration, effort, and dedication, but it's going to make you achieve your personal best."

Self-mastery has a lot of definitions, but I think of it as a process of achieving the greatest possible balance between your body and your mind. It's an intensely personal practice of gaining control so you can operate efficiently and effectively, allowing you to move forward in life. Self-mastery is like one of John's races: it takes discipline and training, and it tests your whole being, but when you become skilled at it, it is the best feeling in the world.

Chewing your food till it becomes a liquid is self-mastery in its most fundamental form because it connects your brain and gut and puts them in full harmony. Typically, these two organs aren't in sync, reacting at different rates to the presence of food. When you begin eating, your adrenal system releases a hormone called *ghrelin*—also known as "the hunger hormone"—but it takes a full twenty minutes for ghrelin to circulate in your bloodstream and reach your brain. Until it gets there, your body has no idea it shouldn't be hungry. So, if you wolf down food without pausing to chew, you will eat more and more and more, believing you're still hungry. With every bite, you literally throw your body off balance.

The negative effects of this imbalance are backed up by science. In 2013, researchers at the University of Birmingham (in England, not Alabama) divided forty-three people into two groups and tested them to see how different rates of mastication impacted their desire to eat. One group consumed a meal at their normal speed and the other chewed each bite for thirty seconds. Two hours after eating, the test subjects were offered bowls of candy. The people who chewed their food for thirty seconds took fewer candies than those who ate faster, suggesting that spending more time with each mouthful of food prevents you from wanting to snack later in the day.

What happens when you snack more? Your blood sugar spikes and you gain weight. Being able to *resist* that urge to snack—and making it easier to maintain a healthy weight—gives you a wonderful feeling of control. It's like you've finally grasped the way to allow your body to hum along in synergy, with no calorie wasted or consumed mindlessly. As you master the rate at which you chew, you start to notice what your body really needs. Is it actually hunger or is your mind just playing tricks on you?

Entrepreneur and noted speaker Sandeep Maheshwari spoke about this exact concept in a *TED Talk* that I absolutely love. He said that after about three weeks of chewing his food thirty-two times (a number whose significance I'll talk about later), he began noticing a difference between his *emotional* hunger and *physical* hunger. When he gave his brain the time it needed to register that his belly was full, he became conscious of his eating habits, and he stopped eating simply because he still had food on his plate. He took back the power that food had over his brain, and that allowed him to master his body and lose inches and pounds.

The Healing Power of Chewing

Chewing your food until it's liquid holds the power to heal your body and boost your immune system. I've already talked about how breaking your food into smaller, more digestible bites before swallowing helps your stomach absorb more nutrients, but I'd like to focus in on one of the most important nutrients for cellular health: protein.

Proteins are found in all kinds of foods from leafy, green vegetables to animal protein to nuts, seeds, and beans. Made up of chains of amino acids, proteins help cells grow, repair, and heal. They also provide structure to cells and tissues, carry essential nutrients within the blood, regulate hormonal responses, and help break down other nutrients. When we don't chew our food well enough, proteins land in the stomach in large chunks. Because your stomach acid and digestive enzymes only work on the surface area of food, they don't get access to as much of this protein as they could. Like so many health issues, the negative results are cumulative: with fewer proteins to metabolize, cells and tissues begin to break down. With fewer digested proteins, these damaged cells and tissues can't be repaired. Your skin, for example, is made up of proteins called *keratin* and *elastin*, so it might start to dull, sag, and wrinkle. Basically, without sufficient protein, negative results literally reveal themselves on your face.

When you gulp food down quickly, you also swallow more air than you would if you ate slowly. Your stomach and intestinal tract fill up with air, leading to bloating, distention, hiccups, acid reflux, heartburn, and gas pain. You may have experienced an extreme version of this if you've ever been startled and swallowed a mouthful of food suddenly. You feel like there's something lodged in your throat, then your esophagus, then down toward your diaphragm. The digestive acid in your stomach bubbles up, causing heartburn all the way up to your throat. This isn't just because food is stuck. There's too much air there, too, which throws your digestive system off balance.

Finally, improperly chewed food also leads to an unhealthy overgrowth of intestinal bacteria in your small intestine. This condition is called *small intestinal bacterial overgrowth*, or SIBO. When more undigested food parts pass through your stomach into your small intestine, digestion slows down, and the bacteria in this organ go into overdrive, multiplying faster than they should in an effort to tackle digestion. You may then develop flatulence, bloating, constipation, cramps, or diarrhea.

Do I Really Need to Chew My Food Thirty-Two Times?

Definitely not. Thirty-two is not a magic number, so don't worry if you only chew twenty-five or twenty-six times. Just chew your food until it's liquid as often as you can and remember to be patient. Sandeep Maheshwari said he had to stick with this step for three weeks to see real results, but when he did, they were *powerful*.

The idea of chewing thirty-two times goes back to the late 1800s, when a food writer named Horace Fletcher decided he wanted to lose weight. He read an article that said each of the thirty-two human teeth should be assigned its own bite, so he put the idea into practice. He lost sixty-five pounds and was so excited he started traveling around the country preaching the gospel of mastication.

Horace Fletcher built up a significant following over the years, and eventually became a millionaire. One of his mottoes was "Nature will castigate those who don't masticate," but I don't subscribe to that theory. The fear of punishment isn't motivating. Your progress through Liquids till Lunch, or any kind of health or wellness program, should be enjoyable and motivating, not a pressure cooker. I'm lucky if I can chew each bite twenty times, and I'm proud of that amount! Besides, chewing one's food is by

MOVE FORWARD EVERY DAY

If you have a mild intolerance to certain foods, yet you can't *imagine* your life without them, try chewing your food till it's liquid to see if that clears up your problems. Your body's inflammatory response to these foods is an immune reaction to a perceived foreign substance entering the bloodstream. In fact, those "foreign substances" may be food particles that are simply too large for your cells to assimilate. If you love bread, but it tends to make your face flushed (an inflammatory response), chewing till the bread particles are liquid will make digestion easier and may prevent the immune reaction.

Please bear in mind I am referring to mild intolerances, *not* food allergies. Always check with your doctor before doing this or if you have questions or concerns.

far the hardest action for most people to do, so you shouldn't live in fear of failure. In Liquids till Lunch, there is *no* failure. Being kind to yourself and focusing on the positive progress you're making is the key to moving forward.

What I take from the number "thirty-two" is the symbolic idea that your mouth—the first entry point in the wonderful journey that is eating and digestion—should derive fulfillment from the work it's doing. Your mouth is underappreciated, and that needs to change. There's great power in pleasure, and food should bring contentment to every part of you.

Chewing and the Pleasure of Food

When we gulp down our food mindlessly, we miss a great deal. We lose the connection our tongues make between the feel and texture of food, and we don't notice the subtle flavors that different ingredients bring. Our noses lose the ability to determine whether we actually crave something, letting our eyes trick us into thinking we're hungry simply because there's food on our plate. Being conscious about chewing and eating roots us to the present, connects us with the people with whom we're sharing our meals, and brings awareness to everything that makes food what it is and all that we appreciate about it.

I became deeply aware of the delicate nuances of food when I went to culinary school a few years after my mom's recovery, during the spring of 2016. I was so inspired by how meals made from fresh, high-quality ingredients had helped my mother's healing that I enrolled at the Institute of Culinary Education (ICE) in Manhattan, a six-month program that's known as one of the top five most competitive culinary schools in the world.

I wasn't your average student there. Not only was I the oldest in my class, but I was also keeping kosher. On top of this, I was eating a gluten-free, dairy-free, mostly plant-based diet. In kosher cooking, meats must be sourced, butchered, and prepared in a precise way; you can't mix meat and dairy; specific ingredients

MOVE FORWARD EVERY DAY

We all sneak in extra meals sometimes. Whether it's a small snack or a plate of leftover dinner with a side of apple pie, "cheating" is totally normal. If you do indulge in a recreational meal (a term I prefer over "cheat meal"), be sure to chew it till it's liquid. You'll absorb all the nutrients that way, keep your energy up, and have fewer unpleasant side effects like gas, bloating, and acid reflux.

aren't permitted; and utensils and dishes for meat and dairy are kept and used separately. ICE wasn't kosher, so I couldn't risk tasting the food I'd cooked because I'd break kosher law if I did.

Most of you understand how central tasting is to meal preparation. If a chef needs to know whether what they're cooking needs a pinch of salt or a dash of something else, they'll dip a spoon into the pot and sample it. Then they'll add the specific ingredient, mix it up a little, grab a new spoon, and taste it again. In order to keep kosher, I wasn't going to be able to do that—*ever*.

Each chef-in-training cooked about six or seven dishes a day, and then our instructors—who were as strict as drill sergeants—sampled them and gave us grades on a 1 to 10 scale. Their feedback was usually brutal, and I was shocked when they praised something I'd made. At the end of the six-month program, all our grades would be tallied up and the faculty and students would cast votes for the Top Toque Award (Top Chef).

The day of the award ceremony, my classmates and I were full of anticipation. We'd spent six months hearing our instructors yell at the top of their lungs, rushing from one end of the kitchen to another, washing dishes till our skin peeled, and heading home reeking of onions and garlic. It had been the hardest unpaid job of my life, and I'd done this on top of running my vitamin business. Now it was time for the Top Toque Award.

I know it might be hard to believe, but even though I never tasted a bite of anything I cooked, I won.

You're probably wondering, *How the heck did you do that, MaryRuth?* It wasn't easy, but I perfected my recipes by using my sense of smell. I drew the aroma of my dish up into my nose, dropped it all the way on the back of my tongue, and savored it slowly, noticing the subtleties of the flavors, the ingredients, and the spice. Just by sniffing, I could concentrate on the rich, complex flavors of the food.

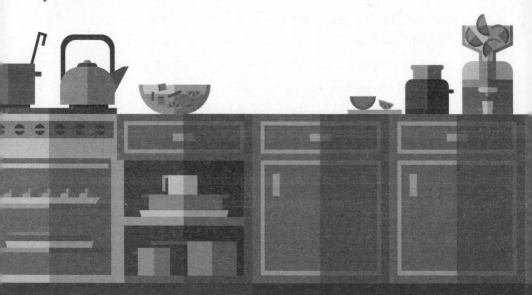

I know smell and taste aren't identical, but the process of savoring the details of food is much the same. When you chew your food slowly, you focus on it. You relish its texture. You appreciate its quality. The top sommeliers in the world treat wine in a similar way. When they taste a wine, they sniff it, twirl their glass to open it up a bit, sip it, and allow it to ripple and roll over their tongues. Then, they don't swallow it. Instead, they spit the wine out, allowing the memory of the flavor not to be tarnished by an alcohol buzz. To experience true, unbridled enjoyment of food, you don't have to swallow it right away. You can sample it, taste it, chew it slowly, and enjoy it. Food can be *bliss*, not just a means to fill you up.

Chewing and Mindfulness

When I was first starting out in my practice, I had a client named Jane who was planning her wedding. It wasn't a fancy ceremony at an expensive restaurant with a $10,000 dress like you'd see on *Say Yes to the Dress*, but it was all Jane had ever wanted. Her arm linked through her dad's, she'd walk down the aisle in the church she went to as a child, then have a delicious buffet-style dinner under a tent in her backyard. Her little sister would be her maid of honor, a local band would play some oldies, and she'd wear her mom's wedding dress.

I adored Jane's energy and excitement. I was thrilled that she'd met a man who loved her deeply, respected the amazing career she'd built, and wanted nothing more than to spend his life with her. Her wedding was going to be a day she'd dreamed about since she was a little girl—but only if she could catch her breath and not feel overwhelmed.

Jane was what Harriet Lerner called in her bestselling book *The Dance of Anger* an "overfunctioner." In times of crisis, her hypermeticulous, ultraorganized nature took over. Sure, her wedding was supposedly simple, but Jane filled it with details and tasks that made it complicated. She leaned into the wedding stress with a to-do list ten miles long and a call sheet that would occupy her half the day. When Jane's divorced parents started fighting about the guest list, Jane jumped in to try to navigate their communication problems. When her florist called saying that some of the flowers she'd sourced might be more expensive than the budget allowed, Jane redesigned all the bouquets and table arrangements herself. And when her notoriously unreliable best friend from college announced he'd broken up with his girlfriend, and could she please seat him at the table with all the single girls, Jane redid the table seating rather than tell him it was too late.

Jane had been seeing me for about four months before her wedding to help her lose weight and she'd been very successful. But in the past three weeks, she'd developed gas, indigestion, and constipation. I was sure these digestive problems weren't helped by her stress level, but I wanted to see exactly how the food and times she was eating affected her body. I asked her to text me a list of her meals every day for one week, indicating where she ate them and just how long it took for her to finish them. I was not surprised *at all* when I saw her first day's results:

MONDAY BREAKFAST: Cappuccino, banana, bowl of whole-grain cereal with milk. Ate it in four and a half minutes while checking emails and unloading the dishwasher.

MOVE FORWARD EVERY DAY

If you're finding it next to impossible to chew your food until it's liquid, try these strategies, which will force you to slow down and become mindful.

- CUT YOUR FOOD INTO SMALLER BITES. You'll have to chew less if your food portions are smaller. Let your fork and knife do the work so your mouth doesn't have to.

- EAT ONLY AT A TABLE. When you're eating on the run or in front of the television or computer, it's hard to focus. Sitting at a table is a signal that it's mealtime, so your brain can focus on the food in front of you.

MIDMORNING SNACK: Half a bowl of nuts sitting at my desk checking emails. Four minutes.

LUNCH: Hummus tahini salad from Sweetgreen. Ate in five minutes sitting in a meeting.

AFTERNOON SNACK: Two blueberry muffins and hot tea. Eaten during a meeting. Three minutes.

DINNER: Roasted chicken, rice, broccoli, two glasses of wine, and piece of cake leftover from an office party. Ate in eight minutes watching TV.

- TRY CHOPSTICKS. Unless you grew up using chopsticks, they're typically harder to eat with than western utensils. Chopsticks will slow your food consumption down and force you to take smaller bites (because they pick up less food than forks or spoons).

- MULTITASK. If you're a busy parent with young children, try sitting with them while they're playing and chew your food as you watch them. I sometimes even clean my children's highchairs while I'm chewing. While this task may sound like a distraction, I have practiced it for a while, and now it works for me. Ultimately, being able to enjoy my lunch and clean up after my children at the same time reduces my stress.

Jane was inhaling her food while standing up, walking around, checking emails, and multitasking. When there was food on her plate, she was avoiding becoming mindful, focusing on the physical act of feeding herself, or chewing thoroughly.

I firmly believe that the essence of self-care involves slowing down and becoming conscious of the present moment. Jane didn't necessarily need to appreciate every bite of her salad, but I knew she was desperate for a deliberate, concerted way to stop moving for more than a few minutes. Jane had never been a big fan of meditation—*My mind goes crazy when I just sit there!*—so I suggested another mindfulness exercise: during every meal, she could sit at a table with her feet on the floor. There could be no television and no iPhone, though background music was fine. Then, she should eat her meal slowly, chewing every bite until it became liquid.

Within a few weeks, Jane was delighted to discover that when she sat down at her dining room table and chewed her food deliberately, her digestive problems improved. She also started to develop creative ideas. She realized who she could introduce to her single college friend, she dreamed up a big marketing idea for her company, and she drafted a script of what she could tell her mom and dad so they'd stop bickering. Her mindfulness wasn't about quieting down her overfunctioning brain, but about giving it a chance to focus. Mindfulness was not meditation; it was concentrated, slowed-down self-care. Jane had never carved out that time till she forced herself to stop and chew her food, and it was a revelation to her.

3.

Drink Half
Your Body Weight
in Ounces of Water

For example: a person who weighs
120 lbs. would drink 60 oz. of water.

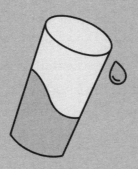

Water is life. From the oceans to the groundwater to the atmosphere to the glaciers, it covers 71 percent of the Earth, providing nourishment to every living thing. Water makes up around 50 to 60 percent of the human body and is the main component of every single one of your organs. It regulates body temperature, flushes out waste, facilitates the digestive processes, helps carry oxygen and essential nutrients to the cells, strengthens your muscles, lubricates your joints, and so much more. Water is so important that when some people don't drink it, they die in three to five days. Think about how fast that is. Now contrast that to the fact that you can live a full *three weeks*—and probably longer—without food.

Even if you're barely active, your body is using the water in its cells. For example, you lose a total of seven cups of water a day just by exhaling and urinating. I promise you'll be shocked if you measure how much that is. Seven cups of water poured into pint glasses is almost four *full* glasses! And you did next to nothing to lose that.

Drinking half your body weight in ounces of water every day is my rule of thumb for good health that reaches all the way down to the cellular level. I know you've all heard the recommendation that eight eight-ounce glasses of water are all you need, but that number doesn't account for how big (or small) you are. A 240-pound professional football quarterback clearly needs more water than a 100-pound high school student.

Drinking enough water every day is an absolute *must*. While there are other actions you can let slide for a day or a week, you cannot, under any circumstances, drink less water than you need. Have I skipped getting sunshine one day? Yes. Have I forgotten to chew my food till it becomes liquid? For sure, especially when I'm rushing through dinner with my children. Have I eaten solid food for breakfast? Of course! I love to cook and eat. But if you neglect drinking half your body weight in ounces of water during the day, you will *really* feel it.

Pain Now or Pain Later

Patricia was a sixty-five-year-old woman who'd just retired after a thirty-five-year career teaching high school English. She had worked hard every single day, creating classes and assignments that her students loved, meeting after hours with those who needed a little extra support, and then coming home to a wonderful husband she'd married right after college. She was the picture of health and happiness in most areas of her life, but she had two big related problems: constant urinary tract infections and constipation. Patricia was from a generation that drank coffee all day long, and she always made a huge pot in the small kitchen at her school. Then she spent every break between classes running back and forth to pour herself a new cup or start a fresh pot.

When Patricia walked into my office, I was shocked that she was only sixty-five. She looked at least seventy-five. Her cheeks were sunken, her eyes had dark circles under them, and her skin was lined with deep wrinkles. Patricia had a huge smile on her face and a spring in her step, so she didn't seem unhappy. But I kept wondering, *Why does she look like she's had the world's hardest life?*

I always ask my clients to complete a written or verbal questionnaire before they come in, and because of that I knew Patricia wasn't a smoker, which would have caused her skin to turn grayish. I also knew she didn't lack for sleep, which might have contributed to the circles under her eyes. I decided to dig a little deeper when we met face-to-face.

"Patricia," I asked, "on average, how much water do you drink a day?"

She paused, then looked down at the cup of coffee she had in her hand. "Two at breakfast and maybe four throughout the day . . . ?" she said, the end of the sentence turning into a question. "I know, I know," she sighed. "I need to drink more water."

In many studies, drinking coffee is actually tied to lower rates of Parkinson's and Alzheimer's, which may be a real benefit. However, coffee acts as a diuretic (leading to increased urination), and that was causing Patricia to be chronically dehydrated. Without sufficient water, Patricia's urinary tract wasn't flushing out properly, allowing bacteria to overgrow. This led to infections. Without enough water in her colon, stools struggled to move along, and that made her constipated.

On a cellular level, Patricia's behavior was impacting not only her appearance but also her ability to function. Water is the building block of our cells, making up about 70 percent of their mass. It gives cells their form and structure the same way air gives a balloon its shape. Without enough water, that same cell loses strength and structure. On the other hand, hydrated cells swell, allowing your skin to plump up. Your complexion then looks firmer, smoother, and less saggy and hollowed out. A hydrated cell flows smoothly and freely through your blood, giving you a natural, dewy glow.

Drinking water is a positive choice with effects that are beneficial immediately *and* over time. There is just no substitute for water. It is a life-giving force on a cellular level, and you need it in abundance every single day if you want to gain any momentum in your life. Patricia was not going to be able to step into a happy retirement with her husband if she struggled with painful, debilitating UTIs every month. She was not going to radiate an image of herself as the smart, capable person I knew she was if she lacked energy and looked older than her actual age.

I always try to focus on the positive—whether it's with my clients, customers, or employees; at home with my husband and children; or out and about in the world running errands, working out, or just having fun. When you've suffered the kinds of devastating losses I have, dwelling on the negative can drag you down and keep you there. You can't change the painful things that have happened to you, so I think it's counterproductive to focus on them to the exclusion of all else. True optimism is believing that life *can* get better, that you can move forward, and that you have the tools to deal with the hardships that will inevitably come your way. A positive outlook is truly motivating and can create a powerful momentum in your life.

But I don't think you should live your life with blinders on, believing that bad things won't happen to you simply because you're so upbeat. The unhealthy choices you make now *will* circle back to you, and there are consequences to unhealthy or destructive behaviors. These negative consequences don't need to happen months or years later, either—like smoking or doing hard drugs. Their results are often immediate. You can choose pain now or pain later, so why not make a choice to tackle a problem today rather than letting it linger and get worse?

MOVE FORWARD EVERY DAY

Flying can be incredibly dehydrating because the pressurized air pulled in from *outside* the plane is very dry. Air at high altitudes doesn't hold as much water vapor as does air near the ground, and that low humidity causes moisture to evaporate from your body quickly. Fill up a water bottle before you board, drink as much of it as you can, then ask the flight attendant to fill it up again after you take off. Always choose an aisle seat, if possible, to make it easier for you to gain access to the lavatory.

While quitting her bad coffee habit wasn't necessarily painful, it was uncomfortable and unpleasant, so Patricia had put it off for years. She chose pain later rather than pain now, and that delay only made her quality of life worse. But when she finally made the choice to help herself, she found out—much to her surprise—that substituting water for coffee wasn't too bad. Within a week, she was down to two cups in the morning and she drank sixty ounces of filtered water the rest of the day. Patricia made a "pain now" decision that guaranteed healthy returns, and she enjoyed a happy, restorative retirement because of it.

The Effects Are Cumulative

Imagine this scenario: You weigh exactly one hundred twenty pounds and are moderately active and in good health. You need to drink sixty ounces of water daily, but, on any given day, you only take in fifty. You may *think* you're doing fine; after all, fifty is close to sixty, right? Yes, but your body doesn't know that. Hidden away from you, deep inside your organ systems, these lost ounces stack up like a pile of dirty laundry, and over the days and weeks, the consequences are cumulative.

If your doctor tested your blood, their diagnostic criteria might not label you as dehydrated, but the cascade of negative health effects happening on the cellular level prove that you are *subclinically* dehydrated—or at an early stage of dehydration. What does this mean? A subclinical diagnosis means that all the signs point to something being wrong, but it doesn't tick off all the boxes and number levels that the medical establishment has set up. So no matter what your test results say, within your body, your cells are just not hydrated at an optimal level. One negative cellular function will lead to another, and that's going to cause problems that are tough to reverse. Your brain will become foggier, and you'll start to slip behind on tasks you should have accomplished. Your urine will become more concentrated, and your kidneys won't function as efficiently. Tiny crystals will grow into stones, and, day by day, those stones will get bigger, then bigger. With each and every ounce of water you skip, you'll set yourself back. And with each passing day, you will struggle more and more to get by.

Let's look a little closer at some of these cumulative health issues. Plasma is the yellowish part of blood that holds blood cells and carries protein, salt, enzymes, and other critical nutrients. Plasma is 95 percent water, and even if you're just subclinically dehydrated, your plasma will thicken, causing your overall blood volume to drop. Think of it like a dry, dirty creek after a few days of no rain. It's sludgy, stale, and stagnant, and there may be dead leaves and sticks struggling to make their way through it. But since you have less of this thick liquid trying to pass through your veins, your cardiovascular system slows down, using less pressure to pump. As your blood pressure drops, you might become dizzy, weak, tired, or experience blurry vision. Your skin might become cold and clammy, and you might even become depressed. All because you drank ten ounces less water than you needed during the day!

Now let's look at your brain. The brain holds on to water like a sponge. When you take in less water than you should, your brain begins to shrink and pull back from your skull. Sound uncomfortable? Well, it is. Your head begins to ache, throb, or pound, a feeling anyone who's ever had a hangover knows. When you drink too much, you rob your body of water because you eliminate so much of it as urine. The pain you feel in your head after a night of too much drinking is partially the result of dehydration, and if you take in even one glass of water, you'll probably start to feel some relief. Your brain will hydrate and plump up again, and that nasty throb will morph into a low-level ache.

Not enough water can affect your mood, exhaustion level, and alertness, too. A 2014 study looked at two groups of people, one which was great at drinking water, and the other that was the opposite. The researchers gave the high-volume drinkers less water and the low-volume drinkers more water over the course of three days. The people who got less water reported a decrease in happiness, calmness, and energy, while those who got more water said their mood and energy level were better than they had been before. The results were definitive: less water means an unhappier, less vibrant you.

Finally, the kidneys function more efficiently when there's enough water in the body. The kidneys are responsible for filtering waste out of the blood and maintaining the body's fluid balance, and if they don't have sufficient water with which to work, they produce darker, more concentrated urine. This is hard work for them, like squeezing an old, dry lemon rather than one that's plump and juicy. Over days and weeks without enough water, kidney tissues wear down and, in addition to urine, they begin to form stones (mentioned earlier). I don't need to tell you that is something that we all desperately want to avoid if possible.

Rest assured, preventing all this trauma and turning around many of your problems is only a glass of water away!

MOVE FORWARD EVERY DAY

When I was growing up, there were three kinds of water: sparkling, tap, and bottled. If you really searched, you could also buy seltzer water with lemon or lime. Now you can find every flavor under the sun, from *pamplemousse* (that's *grapefruit* in French) to "unicorn kisses" (which tastes a little like watermelon). The *Wall Street Journal* published findings that said that 20 percent of people don't like the taste of plain water, so all these flavors are ultimately a good thing if they help people hydrate. But are they healthy? I'm not a huge fan of artificial flavorings because putting chemicals in your body isn't great for you. So if you drink flavored water, try to search for those flavored with "fruit essence," which is a naturally derived oil from the skin of a fruit. Better yet, flavor your own water with

The Healing Magic of Water

Enough about all the bad things that happen when you don't drink water. Water holds power because it's a simple thing that can radically and quickly change your life for the better. The payback it delivers can be incredibly positive, so let's focus on the good stuff.

Water is one of the best ways to boost your immunity. As much as a good diet and healthy behaviors, such as exercise and stress management, can help your body fight any number of

a splash of fruit juice or stevia. A little goes a long way, so you only need a few drops.

My stance is that noncarbonated water is always better than carbonated because the bubbles can cause internal gas pressure that can lead to bloating, indigestion, or even headaches. But do your best and start wherever you need to. Hydration is the most important thing.

Because coconut, cactus, and other alternative waters may have sugar or be high in calories, don't drink these to the exclusion of all else. But if you like having a glass or two a day to break up your routine, that's fine! Just know that the research is mixed as to whether they hydrate as well as water—some studies say they hydrate better, while others say they don't. When in doubt, stick to plain water.

health problems, drinking half your body weight in ounces of water daily can do that and then some.

The immune system is a complex and interconnected network comprised of your spleen, bone marrow, thymus, lymph and lymphatic vessels, and more. When a virus, bacteria, or allergen (like pollen) enters your body, your cells recognize it as a foreign agent. Your white blood cells, which are produced in the bone marrow, travel through the lymphatic system, ultimately attacking the germ or allergen that is attempting to make you sick.

Let's look at lymph, since water is central to it. Lymph is a viscous substance that collects bacteria and germs and carries them to the lymph nodes, where they're destroyed. *Lymph* actually means *water* in Latin, and that's no accident because it's made up of 95 percent water. Unlike the circulatory system, the lymphatic system doesn't have a pump, so it needs help moving the lymph along through your body. You can kickstart this process through exercise or a good massage, but if you don't have enough water flowing through your body, your lymph is going to be stagnant. Think of that mucky stream again. It needs clean, fresh water to keep it moving, and if it doesn't get it, it won't be able to do its job of washing away waste and debris and nourishing the living systems that surround it.

Water can also help your joints tremendously. The joints are made up of a shiny, slippery substance called *articular cartilage*, which is comprised of 60 percent water. This cartilage contains a substance called *synovial fluid*, which acts as a lubricant, allowing your bones to move smoothly against each other. If you're dehydrated, your joints will chafe together, causing friction that can aggravate arthritis or a joint injury. If there's too much friction, the joint may become inflamed, causing even more pain. With good hydration, though, the cartilage can stay well lubricated, and you can prevent or reduce inflammation. Even better, water encourages the growth of new cells in the cartilage.

Food, Water, and Balance

A lot of you are convinced that going to extremes is a surefire way to lose weight, get your energy back, or jump-start your life. This may be true; raw food diets, high-protein diets, or juice fasts can be truly nutritious, energizing, and slimming for many people. In the last fifteen years of my life, I've completed one forty-day juice fast—when I consumed only juice—and many shorter fasts. I've seen amazing results in my life because of them. A friend of mine recently did a two-week water fast (meaning he consumed only water), and his skin has never looked so clear or his eyes so bright. He also said he felt fabulous the whole time, with a sense of purpose and fulfillment he'd never had. Just remember: Always check with your doctor before you begin fasting.

We know extreme diets aren't for everyone, and they're not always the magic formula to change your life. I much prefer the gradual, cumulative cellular benefits of Liquids till Lunch rather than fasting. In general, I think the body needs balance, and regularly putting it through a drastic or intense situation can cause real suffering, from exhaustion to extreme hunger to anxiety. You need a *consistent* level of good energy to stay at the top of your game. Good hydration from a range of places can help you achieve that.

Water is your body's great leveler, allowing all its systems to work in harmony. But to achieve balance in the body, water needs to come from the right variety of sources. Straight water—especially filtered water free of impurities—should always be your first tier of hydration. Herbal tea, whose base is entirely made of water, is also fine. Please avoid slipping into the habit of drinking tea rather than water, though, and drink only a cup or two of tea a day.

Raw fruits and vegetables are the second great source of water, and researchers estimate that up to 20 percent of our water intake comes from food. My recommendation is to strike a balance between

MOVE FORWARD EVERY DAY

I know some of you aren't fans of stepping on the scale, and I understand that. But it's important to know your body weight so that you can ensure you're taking in the right amount of water. I recommend weighing yourself at least once a week. Then, find a water bottle you love that you can carry with you to work, in the car, everywhere you go. Know how many ounces it holds and fill it up a few times a day accordingly. Based on my weight, I fill mine up three times—or more if I'm pregnant or nursing and weigh more than I usually do.

water-dense foods (fruits and vegetables) and nutrient-dense foods (potatoes, animal proteins, grains, beans, nuts, and seeds).

The Importance of pH Balance

The pH level of substances is measured on a scale of 0 to 14. Everything below 7 is acidic, and everything above 7 is alkaline. Geologists regularly test the pH of groundwater and drinking water because the acid/alkaline balance is an important measure of pollution; if pH changes dramatically, there may be toxins in your water. Ever hear of the term *acid rain*? It's precipitation with a pH of around 5.6, which has become acidic due to high levels of carbon dioxide emissions from factories and cars.

People who work in the functional medical field—like nutritionists, Ayurvedic practitioners, or health educators like me—have always believed that it's possible for your cells' pH to become too acidic as a result of the foods you put in your body. Scientists and mainstream doctors didn't rally behind this idea until about ten years ago, but now that a few studies have supported it, it's beginning to gain traction with the establishment. Foods with a high-acid load include animal proteins like beef, pork, or poultry; and eggs, beans, and seed oils like canola or peanut oil. When you eat them, your body releases acid into the bloodstream. If your pH is chronically high, you suffer from a disorder called *acidosis*. Acidosis increases your likelihood of developing metabolic syndrome, cancer, osteoporosis, and kidney stones.

MOVE FORWARD EVERY DAY

Maintaining a healthy weight by eating a nutritious, balanced diet is important for a great number of reasons, but I believe that you should never allow yourself to get overly hungry. If you're famished, you are not in a place to make healthy decisions that will move you in a positive direction. Secondly, excessive hunger may drive you to overeat or snack too much, and that will undo all the good work you've done. So, when you hit the salad bar, include a bit of quinoa and avocado with your red pepper, lettuce, and shaved carrots. This nutrient-dense and water-dense balance will give you key nutrients and make you feel full.

The body strives for balance, so it deals with excessive acid in your bloodstream through respiration—when you breathe out carbon dioxide, you lower your pH—and through your kidneys. When the kidneys filter out sulfate, phosphate, urate, chloride, calcium, and ammonium ions, they help level out your body's pH. If your pH is chronically acidic, you may develop kidney stones. Research shows that taking potassium and magnesium citrate supplements can prevent and reverse the formation of these stones, but there's one other thing that can help: water. The positive effects of drinking water are immediate *and* cumulative. Water dilutes the minerals in your kidneys that may lead to stones. Fewer stones means the kidneys can work efficiently and stay strong. Strong, functional kidneys can help ease you gracefully through the aging process.

In the past few years, alkaline water has become hugely popular because of claims that it can help regulate pH. Many people question this because there are no rigorous studies to back it up, but I'm a huge fan for personal reasons. I suffered terrible morning sickness throughout my pregnancies, and alkaline water always helped with my nausea. I've also seen a few studies that show alkaline water can assist with acid reflux, high blood pressure, diabetes, high cholesterol, and blood viscosity. I firmly believe that what works for you may not work for someone else, so if alkaline water helps you, go for it. But don't drink it to the exclusion of all else. Water with a pH of 8 or 9—which is what alkaline water holds—does not exist in nature in abundance, so you have to be delicate with it. The best long-term approach to good health is one that's steady, stable, and natural, so if it's easy for you to find, drink one glass or bottle of alkaline water daily in combination with other types of water.

Scheduling Creates Positive Momentum

As I said earlier, one of my mottoes is "structure creates freedom." Because I run a company with over seventy employees for whom I feel tremendous personal responsibility (not to mention a lot of love) and have a young family that needs every bit of me, my life is overwhelming in its best moments. On a Sunday night, I have a to-do list for the week a mile long, and it would be super easy for me to feel overwhelmed and powerless. Sometimes I do! But I carefully create—then live, breathe, and act on—a life of positive structure, and it gives me so much freedom. Rather than feeling trapped or stuck, I know exactly what I'm facing and when I'm going to have to deal with it, and that empowers me. I understand that through my program, within a twenty-four-hour period I will execute micro actions that will consistently, yet gradually, create a powerful momentum that pushes me forward and changes the macro landscape of my life. If something happens that makes my momentum go downhill—my son gets sick, my car breaks down, or, God forbid, anything worse—I can return to that structure because I know it's safe. Just putting myself in that positive place when the time is right will heal me and point me back in the right direction.

Let's narrow this concept down even more and talk about scheduling. I am a total scheduler. By Monday morning, I know what my week is going to look like down to the hour, and that's exactly how I like it. You might not be as type A as me, and that's totally fine. But I do feel that there's a real comfort that comes with a certain degree of scheduling—meaning one that doesn't feel restrictive—because it can be such a powerful force in healing your body and giving you energetic momentum.

Your water intake is an easily scheduled micro action that can change the macro landscape of your body and support all the good you're doing in life. After you wake up, drink a glass of water. Before you go to work, drink another. Set an alarm every hour, and then drink a glass when the alarm goes off. If you wait until you're thirsty, your cells will have already shrunken enough to send a signal to your brain telling you to drink. You will have tackled your problem too late, and the effects will be felt in your kidneys, your brain, your cells, your skin, and more. Who wants that negative momentum? No one.

You should also stop drinking water fifteen minutes before you eat. Most of us wash our food down with liquid, but since my program teaches you to chew your food till it's liquid (and I hope you're going to try it!) there's no need for that. Some people have theorized that digestive enzymes won't be able to reach food if there's too much water in your stomach, but that's not true. Water also won't dilute your digestive acid. The reason I recommend stopping your water intake fifteen minutes before you eat is because even a moderate amount of water in combination with food can cause gas and bloating. It can also make you feel full, which will trick your

MOVE FORWARD EVERY DAY

If you're drinking half your body weight in ounces of water during the day, you should be going to the bathroom at least once an hour. If you're urinating less often than that, you're either not drinking enough, or you're losing more water than average through sweating. If you exercise a lot and find that's the case, simply take in more water before and after you work out.

brain into believing you don't need to eat more. You might think this is a good thing if you're try- ing to lose weight but, during meals, you should always be aware of how much food you need to fill yourself up and keep your body in balance.

I don't start drinking water again until an hour after I eat for the same reason. I want to understand the sensation of being full and not assume that I ate too much. Even though it takes four to five hours for food to leave your stomach and enter your small intestine, an hour is a reasonable amount of time for your stomach to settle and give you a sense of whether you've con- sumed enough.

Healing Through Scheduled Repetition

As you know, the body has a powerful system of circadian rhythms that tell it when to expect food. Scheduled eating cre- ates intelligence within the cells, then soothes and balances them. It stands to reason that scheduled water intake is no different. Water cleanses, lubricates, and relaxes your body whether you are drinking it, bathing in it, or swimming through it. It heals at the most fundamental level, so if you pair it up with a schedule, I can promise you the health-restoring power will multiply tenfold.

In exceedingly stressful times, our bodies surge with adrena- line, bracing us for a crisis that has either happened or is about to happen. In what's known as the *fight-or-flight response*, our shoulders tense, hearts race, and blood pressure rises. These times of intense stress can go on and on and on—think of your quarantine during the COVID-19 pandemic, when a loved one was sick, or when you were having relationship issues. You might feel intense adrenaline when something good happens, too, like when you start a new job or plan a party or your wedding. Your body is amped up, on edge, and ready to go. That much adrenaline running through

MOVE FORWARD EVERY DAY

Ayurvedic and Chinese medicine practitioners have claimed for years that drinking warm or room temperature water is better for you than cold water. They say that cold water constricts blood vessels in the stomach and small intestine, slows enzyme secretion (which hinders good digestion), and causes lymph to stagnate. While there's not much research to support these claims, warm water does help clear your nasal passages and helps blood flow more quickly to your intestines (because it widens the blood vessels). I've also found that, like a bowl of vegetable soup or a mug of herbal tea, it relaxes me. The warmth fills my belly, giving me a sense of being fully present. So, while drinking cold water may not hurt you, why not try room-temperature water? You might discover you really love it—and so might your body.

your system over the long term is *exhausting*, and when you can't take the pressure anymore, you will crash.

Bessel van der Kolk, the *New York Times* bestselling author of *The Body Keeps the Score: Brain, Mind, and Body in the Healing of Trauma*, spoke recently about what happens to you while you brace for the impact of a trauma. In an intimidating, unpredictable situation, you feel out of control and unable to do anything. Your mind and body often freeze up like a deer in headlights, and you may stay up all night with insomnia, spend hours glued to the TV, or sit at your kitchen table chain-smoking cigarettes or downing glass after glass of wine. In order to counter this unpredictability, Dr. van der Kolk says that one of the best possible things you can do to take care of yourself is to set a strict schedule. Schedules give your body a sense of regularity, relaxing it into the notion that life is, in fact, normal. If your body knows what to expect, it will signal to your mind to stop panicking. Your body will channel the idea that the chaos is bearable, and that you can handle it with just a little bit of self-care.

Drinking water on a predictable schedule and in abundance can be essential to that healing. Water is a radical force for good, creating a powerful momentum that cannot be understated. Out of all the actions in my program, it's the one with the most immediate positive impact. Don't you want to make that great energy a regular, essential part of your routine? I promise you, it's totally worth it.

4.

Portion Control

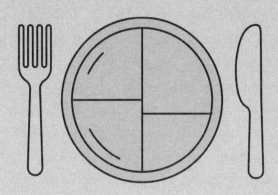

You are what you eat" is a popular old saying. The truth is that you are what you *digest*. The simple acts of eating and digestion are natural, cellular processes that have transformative effects on your whole being. The three Krispy Kreme donuts you gobbled up during your breakfast meeting broke down in your mouth and stomach, were absorbed into your small intestine, and then powered your cells through a series of chemical processes. Every organ, tissue, and fluid in your body is made up of cells, and every action and reaction within your body doesn't exist without the work they do. Just as plants harness the energy of sunshine to grow, flower, and bloom, those Krispy Kremes produced dramatic cellular and chemical effects on your body's processes and actions, allowing you to become—in big and small ways—a different person than you were before you ate them.

The issue is: Don't we all want to be healthier than a donut? Don't we all want to feel more energetic, experience greater mental clarity, and embrace satisfying routines and practices that cause us to move forward every day? Yes, definitely. That's why you have to think very carefully not only about *what* you're putting in your body, but also *how much*. You are nothing more than a bunch of cells that come together to form a bunch of organs, so you have to treat yourself well all the way down to these teeny, tiny building blocks of life. There are few things more beneficial to cellular self-care than portion control.

Portion control is not as straightforward as you might think. Eating the right amount may not be about eating less. Some of you may need to eat more, and some of you may need to sit down for meals at different times. Portion control is a *feeling* and a *way of conducting yourself*. It's an understanding of your body's digestive needs and a sense of when you're full. It's the realization that you have power over your food, rather than the reverse. Your body strives for balance, and when you master the art of portion control, that's what you achieve.

The Notion of Cellular Self-Love

My client, Kate, was a fifty-year-old book editor who was supposed to be at the height of her career. She'd spent her twenties and thirties working her way up at a small, prestigious publishing house, where she'd discovered a handful of literary authors she groomed into critical and commercial successes. With her vision, dedication, and careful editing, her authors won one literary award after another and their books were steady bestsellers.

In her mid-forties, Kate was given her own imprint at a big, cash-rich publishing house, and she brought her bestselling authors with her, instantly establishing herself as the most profitable and glamorous editor in the business. Kate got invited to every cocktail party and gala event in town, and she dressed perfectly in clothes she'd bought off the rack at Saks. Her taste in jewelry was as interesting and artistic as her publishing list, and she kept everyone up on the latest gossip at all the see-and-be-seen lunch spots in Manhattan. At her favorite restaurant—where she always sat in the same seat—the waiter knew her lunch order by heart: Niçoise salad with the egg and potatoes on the side. Sparkling water with a twist of lemon. No dessert—ever.

Kate maintained a healthy weight, but part of her still felt like the chubby bookworm who everyone had made fun of in middle school. It went against all her impulses to make frivolous small talk; she just wanted to run home and curl up in bed with her husband—who'd been her first and only boyfriend—and a book. So when her husband left her for a younger woman, Kate fell into a deep depression. Then another publishing house stole one of her bestselling authors, and her self-esteem fell even more. She felt hopeless, lost, and unable to get over these unbelievable betrayals.

Kate maintained appearances at work, still dressing beautifully and eating the same tiny salad at lunch every day, but when she got home, she *ate*. Her husband wasn't there to see her naked anymore, so she figured, *Who cares?* She ordered double portions from all her favorite take-out places and washed her meals down with a bottle of wine. Then she polished it all off with half a pint of ice cream. By the time she came to see me, she'd put on twenty pounds.

"I don't have a husband or children at home to tell me to stop eating so much," she told me one afternoon as tears streamed down her face. "And, honestly, I just don't care. If I can still dress well and impress everyone at meetings, I can get by."

"But is just 'getting by' enough?" I asked.

"No," she answered, starting to tear up. "But I don't know where to start."

I looked Kate right in the eyes and smiled. "It's going to be okay," I said. "I'm going to help you get back on track by keeping you accountable for what you eat. But I think we need to look a little deeper than what you're ordering from the local Thai restaurant."

Kate's problem wasn't self-awareness; she was crystal clear about the fact that she was overeating to cover up her pain and sense of abandonment—and, conversely, that in the past she'd undereaten to keep up appearances. Plus, understanding yourself is necessary and great, but I'm not sure it always moves you forward—especially when you're as stuck as Kate was. She needed to *act* on her self-awareness, and that required self-love.

Let's look a little more closely at the definition of self-love. While you can think of it as a negative characteristic, like narcissism, that's not what I mean. Self-love is a fundamental appreciation for how precious your body is to your life. It's an understanding that, if you want to move forward every day, you have to value, respect, and care for every single one of your cells and organs. You only have one body, and you owe it everything because it alone allows you to live.

Kate's decision to stuff herself every night reflected how she felt about her life and the space her body inhabited in it. She had beautiful clothes, a perfect manicure, and an expensive haircut, but her view of herself stopped with her looks, her achievements, and the fact that her husband had once loved her. She

MOVE FORWARD EVERY DAY

I love using visualization to help me think differently about my decisions. The concept I'm about to explain to you may sound crazy, but I've used it many times with my clients, and it always clicks with them. Imagine there's something central to your self-care that you find really hard to do. Let's say it's eating the right amount. You love sweets, and the idea of skipping dessert or your morning cinnamon-roll frappuccino sounds unbearable, even if you know eating it will fill you to the point of being uncomfortable. Now, pretend someone said to you, "I will give you a million dollars if you skip that frappuccino tomorrow." You would for sure, absolutely, 100 percent not go to Starbucks. Not only that, but you would be thrilled to wake up, get in the car, and drive two miles out of your way so you wouldn't pass that Starbucks and be tempted. You would make a point to avoid sweets because you were so excited about that million dollars. So, just know that—no matter what you think is holding you back from doing something that will move you forward in life—you have it within yourself to do it. You hold the strength and the power, so don't let your mind trick you into thinking you don't.

didn't understand that how she treated her digestive tract, the way she chewed and drank water, and how much she put on her plate were fundamental parts of her self-care routine. She didn't understand that, in order to love yourself, you have to treat your cells better than you treat your best pair of shoes.

We all know how devastating cancer is on both physical and emotional levels. Even though my mom didn't have cancer, she suffered through two brain tumors and two very serious surgeries to remove them, so I'm empathetic to the fact that the disease is *horrible*. But a lot of patients report positive emotional changes that come out of their cancer treatments or surgeries. Their self-esteem goes up as they start to appreciate the strength of their bodies. Their priorities shift, and they may thank their stomach, breasts, ovary—or whatever organ or body part is suffering—for all the hard work it's done to make their lives possible. If they recover, they stop abusing their bodies through drinking, smoking, or overeating. Those who've lost their hair through chemo may stop coloring it when it grows back because they're so grateful for its natural beauty.

Self-love gives you this clarity of purpose. It shows you how and why to give your body exactly the right amount of food so it can deliver exactly the right amount of energy to power you out of a tough problem—or make a good problem even better. Self-love gives your life momentum, so I urge you to view yourself as more than what appears on the outside. You are also a collection of cells and organs coming together to make one unified, beautiful you.

The Health Benefits of Portion Control

The most obvious negative health effect of overeating is weight gain. If you consistently take in more calories than you burn, and if you consistently have elevated blood-sugar levels from eating too much of the wrong foods, you will store those extra calories as fat. More fat means more weight.

Doctors and health professionals typically measure how much weight is too much for your body through something called the *body mass index*, or BMI. BMI is calculated as:

**(703 × YOUR WEIGHT IN POUNDS)
DIVIDED BY (YOUR HEIGHT IN INCHES SQUARED)**

If you weigh 200 pounds and are five feet, ten inches tall, your BMI would be:

(703 × 200) = 140,600

Divided by (70 squared, or 4,900) = 28.69

A BMI less than 18.5 is considered underweight, while one between 18.5 and 24.9 is normal. From 25 to 29.9 is considered overweight, and any number 30 and over is categorized as obese. Obesity is a major risk factor for any number of diseases including high blood pressure, cardiovascular disease, cancer, liver and kidney disease, diabetes, and—recently—COVID-19. In 2014, researchers aggregated the results of twenty different long-term studies on obesity and concluded that people with a BMI over 40 live on average six and a half years less than those who aren't obese, and extremely obese people—those who have a BMI over 55—live on average fourteen fewer years. In terms of life expectancy, that means obesity is as harmful as smoking. And the heavier you are, the more dangerous than smoking it is.

When I talk about self-love, I want to be clear that I am not implying that people who put on weight or become obese don't love themselves or value their lives. Self-love is a process of becoming aware of your body's needs, not treating it perfectly all the time. I am also not putting down anyone who's struggled to lose weight or is currently on a diet. I just want to urge you to think carefully about your body and obesity's effects on it. Just as with drinking enough water, the choices you make will catch up to you, so I strongly urge you to consider what's best for you and decide accordingly. You can literally lose *years* of your life because of excess weight.

Lack of portion control overtaxes your digestive system as well. When there's more food in your belly than your body is comfortable with, your stomach expands. This expansion puts pressure on your other organs and diminishes their effectiveness. They begin to slow down to conserve energy, causing you to feel tired or sluggish. At the same time, your stomach and the other digestive organs have to secrete additional enzymes and acids in order to metabolize the huge amount of food in your belly, taxing them even further. Plus, all the extra hydrochloric acid in your gut can seep into your esophagus, causing you to develop heartburn.

Overeating can also disrupt the connection between your stomach and your brain. Typically, it takes about twenty minutes for the brain to receive a signal from the neurological tissue at the top of your belly, signaling that it's full. Again, this time delay is why I recommend chewing your food until it becomes liquid; you'll be forced to slow down and give your brain those precious extra minutes to catch up. But research also shows that the delicate tissue on your stomach can malfunction when you consistently overeat, causing your brain to receive irregular messages about being full. In fact, you may never even know you're full, and you'll keep eating and eating and eating. Soon, you'll be packing in so much food that you'll do lasting damage to your digestive system and your waistline. Also, when you overeat you feel less energetic because the energy in your body moves from healing and repair to digestion.

Your metabolism also rises when you overeat. Metabolism is defined as the amount of energy (measured in calories) that's required to keep your body's very basic functions (like brain activity, circulation, and digestion) functioning. If there's a lot of food in your stomach, you need more energy, so your metabolism will go up accordingly. Imagine a campfire that's burning at a slow and steady pace, but you decide to throw a few dry logs and a bunch of old newspaper on it. Guess what happens? Flames begin to rise, smoke billows up and out, and heat and energy radiate in all directions. That's what happens in your stomach when there's too much food, so it's no wonder that overeating may cause you to become hot, sweaty, or dizzy.

Almost everyone consumes too much food on occasion, especially on vacations and holidays. And you might be convinced that if you make up for it the next day or week—by dieting, fasting, or exercising just a little bit more than you normally would—that you'll be fine. Unfortunately, that may not be the case. A significant number of people die on Thanksgiving, Christmas, the day after Christmas, or on New Year's Day. While there are a few theories about why this happens, researchers from the University of Melbourne in Australia recently determined that suicide, car crashes, or other "unnatural" causes aren't to blame. Instead, cardiac deaths spike on those days. What causes heart attacks? It could be the stress of being with your family, but all the evidence points to the fact that people almost always overconsume food on these days.

Finally, research shows that short-term periods of overeating can trigger changes in your body's internal clock. Scientists from Northwestern University recently discovered that mice who were overfed woke up during the night so they could eat more, and these late-night binges caused them to put on massive amounts of weight. Yes, we're human beings, not mice, but the research was so solid, and the effects so definitive, that the scientists were confidently able to conclude that eating sensible portions regulates your circadian rhythms. This, in turn, allows you to sleep better.

Seek Answers That Are Fluid, Not Rigid

This is not a diet book, so I won't give you precise instructions on how many calories you need to consume based on your BMI.

In my years of work with clients, I learned that almost everyone loses weight in different ways. That's because weight loss is a complicated process that involves your activity level, your age, the size of your frame, the quality of food you eat, your lifestyle, and more. For a lot of you, it may be hard to hear that dieting isn't as easy as just eating less food. You might want to give up all control to a program that promises exact results if you do X, Y, and Z, or you may want someone to hold you accountable for every bite you put in your mouth, but that's not how this particular action in my program works. While I'll give you some guidelines about scheduling when you eat—and the effects it will have on your body—I can't tell you exactly what to do and promise you'll have perfect results.

What I will say is: If you form your own structure and routine that make you happy and energized within the framework of your one-of-a-kind life, you will create tremendous freedom for yourself. This freedom feels *amazing*, and you will love owning your success rather than giving up all the credit to someone else. You know what's best for you, and you alone understand what suits your family's needs. I can promise that what works for you is different than what works for some other family. So while I'll give you suggestions, I also believe independence will offer you tremendous power.

In almost anything related to your health, bear in mind that the answers you seek may be fluid and imprecise. That's okay! I've gone through this myself and, to be honest, the flexibility came as a huge relief. I was diagnosed with Lyme disease in 2015 after spending years going from one doctor to another trying to figure out why I had skin rashes all the time and why I kept having miscarriages. Each doctor looked at my symptoms, ran blood tests, and then replied with certainty that they knew exactly what was wrong with me and the exact health protocol I should follow to fix it. That helped a little but not a lot.

I finally went to a functional medicine doctor who listened to me carefully and asked me dozens of questions, not just about my symptoms but also about my diet, habits, and lifestyle. She took blood tests, but when the results came back, she didn't look at their levels and stop there. She combined my results with her clinical observations, realizing that blood tests may not tell the whole story. Often, a doctor needs to string together patients' mysterious symptoms with their test results for a successful diagnosis. Difficult illnesses don't necessarily follow a pattern.

"I think you have Lyme disease," she said the second time we met.

"What should I do?" I asked.

Her answer wasn't what I expected.

"It depends," she said. "You have to listen to your body and be flexible with the protocol and guidelines I'm going to recommend."

Her solution was not rigid. It was not about what was best for most people, it was about what would work for *me*. Yes, she prescribed me some medicine and supplements, recommended a specific diet and a few alternative therapies, and gave me advice about how to alter my lifestyle. But she also suggested the possibility of changing it all if my symptoms didn't get better. She was adaptable and accommodating and, with the freedom and power she'd offered me, I took charge of my health and got better because of it.

With any health modality, I think an inflexible protocol that gives you no freedom is a huge red flag—whether it comes from a doctor, a podcast, or from a health educator like me. You need tips you can mold into your own time management plan because

MOVE FORWARD EVERY DAY

My dad was a master of moderation. I don't think I ever saw him eat or drink so much that he lost control. From his workload to his exercise habits to how he spent his money, he knew how to pace himself, and I believe that's why he achieved so much success in his short forty-two years. My dad told me that if he was invited to a party during law school, he would sit in the library and study till just past the time the party started. Then he'd put down his books and walk into the party an hour and a half late. He said he got so much more work done that way *and* got to enjoy the party. It was a win-win for him. We all love to find balance and the win-wins in our personal lives, so I encourage you to find the right balance for yourself, too.

you understand yourself better than anyone. You know when you're traveling, have a deadline at work, are struggling with an illness, or are otherwise incapable of following a set schedule. You also understand when you're fired up, ready to do anything that will move you forward. With this flexibility, you can create your own structure, and that will give you the breathing room to finally take action and find your zone.

Finding Your Zone

Having children has been one of the best and most eye-opening experiences of my life. Children can be exhausting, but they also have a natural wisdom that makes you stop and think about life totally differently than you did before. Their words and actions are entirely based on instinct, and aren't constrained by the rules that society puts on you as you grow up. The eyes of children are clear and innocent, and it's impossible for them to hold back how they feel, whether it's through crying, dancing, or the five hundred hugs and kisses they give you when you're putting them to bed at night.

Children also know when they've eaten enough, and they have no problem leaving food behind on their plates. "I'm full!" they'll yell, even though they've only had two bites of pasta. Sometimes, they skip dinner entirely or go a full week eating nothing but fruit and almond butter. I know how frustrating this is to parents, and I feel it all the time when my children act this way. But their behavior isn't unnatural or rude. Not finishing your meal is totally, completely natural. The body has biological mechanisms that tell it when it's full, and adults ignore these when they eat too quickly, pig out because they love the taste of something, or worry about looking ungrateful.

It's time to let go of those hang-ups and find your zone so you won't overeat. I can promise you that discovering it is going to take time and practice, but when you get there it will feel completely normal. Going back to that place will feel like second nature, and you won't have a problem putting down your fork in the middle of dessert and saying, "Okay, I'm good now." Just think about how you eat when you're sick. You probably have no problem skipping a meal or leaving half your food on your plate when your body tells you enough is enough. Keep that feeling with you even when you're well. If you're full, you're full, so stop eating.

I don't have a magic formula you can follow to know when you've hit your zone. One major step toward discovering this zone is to remember the times you've overeaten. How did you feel? Heavy, weighted down, tired, guilty, or full of self-loathing? Remember those feelings because those are the sensations you want to avoid. At each meal, keep them in the back of your mind but don't dwell on them. Eating should be a joyful, positive experience, so focus on chewing your food till it's liquid and savoring the quality, texture, and flavor of each bite. But don't lose sight of what's going on in your belly. Your stomach—not your brain or the food on your plate—is what will tell you it's time to stop.

Finding your zone is really about discovering your point of *satisfaction*. Think about that word. Satisfaction is neither joy nor misery; it's a level of contentment that's steady, balanced, and constant. Satisfaction also contains an element of surprise, as if you've exceeded your expectations in a small, pleasant way. You're energized by a tingling, buzzing feeling of "just enough" in your stomach. There's no sense of pressure against your belt or any weight pulling you down. You're just right, and you have the energy and desire to take on the day's tasks.

MOVE FORWARD EVERY DAY

One of the easiest ways to promote good digestion and prevent overeating is to consume your meals from light to heavy. What does that mean? Light foods are raw foods like salad or cut vegetables, which have lots of digestive enzymes. Heavy foods are cooked foods, and they fill you up more. If you eat light foods before heavy foods, your enzymes will start to metabolize food into energy. When you move on to the heavier, cooked foods, your digestive system will be buzzing, and you'll digest smoothly without feeling too much gas pressure or bloating. You also won't be tempted to overeat the heavy foods because the light, water-dense foods will have taken the edge off your hunger.

Oftentimes, the trigger for knowing that you've hit the zone is that you
sit back and pause. Maybe you put
your fork down. Maybe you start a
new conversation. Maybe you excuse
yourself to go to the bathroom. Whatever that moment is, stop and think
about how your body feels. Are you hungry? If so, maybe you haven't finished eating.
Personally, I cannot leave the table still feeling hungry. While it's
entirely up to you, my recommendation is to do the same because
if you don't, you'll probably go back to the table and overeat.

Clients often ask whether being in the zone is the same as
having Eye of the Tiger. It's close, but it's not exactly the same.
There's an intensity to Eye of the Tiger, as if you're prepared to
spring into action. You're slightly on edge, but not in a nervous
way. You're simply focused, invigorated, and *ready*. When you're
in the zone, you're also energized, but it's from the position of
knowing you've done what you need to do for yourself and can
take a moment to enjoy it. You don't have to get up and do anything; you can simply sit back, feel pleasantly full, and realize you
have all that you need to move forward.

The Power of Planning

One of my most memorable clients was a young emergency room
doctor named Sandy. Sandy was one of those people who didn't

feel like she was living her best life if she wasn't on her feet doing *something*, and she'd definitely chosen the right job for that. She worked ten twelve-hour shifts per month, moving from crisis to crisis as she tried to save people from the brink of death. Over the course of each shift, she rarely sat down, and when she returned home she crashed into her bed and slept for ten to twelve hours. On her days off, she'd go running or to spin class, longing for the adrenaline rush she'd experienced in the ER.

Sandy came to me because she'd just turned thirty and thought she needed to start making healthier food choices in her life. She had a tendency to eat on the run, grabbing a few donuts from the break room before she was called off to handle another incoming patient. When she got home, she'd heat up leftovers at 2 a.m. and stuff herself, drink a few glasses of wine, and pass out cold. She loved when people ordered pizza at the hospital because that meant she could eat four or five slices and chat about the events of the shift with her friends.

Sandy honestly had no idea how much she was eating because she rarely looked at what she put on her plate. Food went from hand to mouth while her eyes were glued to the TV or her fellow doctors. Sandy hadn't put on much weight because she exercised the calories off, but she felt, in her words, "yucky and tired."

"I'm not strong," she said. "I'm run-down and bloated all the time. I just want to get up and do something on my days off, but the best I can do is exercise, and even that doesn't energize me. I just crash when I get home and sleep like crazy on my days off. What is going on?"

Just as I did with Naomi—who I talked about in action one—I reached into my desk and pulled out a piece of paper. I drew a circle on it and ticked off twelve lines to make it look like a clock. Then I asked Sandy to map out her mealtimes, estimating when and how much she was eating.

MOVE FORWARD EVERY DAY

Every Sunday and Thursday, I cook a pot of vegetable broth to eat throughout the week, and it has changed my life. This simple soup gives me energy and nourishment and allows me to control my portions by filling me up just enough. It's perfect as a light starter before your heavier entrees, or you can put it in a thermos and sip it in the morning till lunchtime. If noon rolls around and you are way too busy to go pick up lunch, don't worry! You'll have your thermos. I also believe in lunch boxes with ice packs for meals and snacks, so carry those along just in case.

If you google "vegetable broth recipe," there are thousands of suggestions on how to make it. My favorite recipe is on the next page. You can tailor your recipe however you like, making the portions bigger or smaller or throwing in different herbs. Cooking according to your own taste is empowering, so have fun.

When you drink your soup, be sure to swish it around inside your mouth so your salivary enzymes can begin to break down its nutrients. Then sit back and enjoy the energized sense of fullness that means you have hit your zone!

"I don't even know," she answered. "I just eat whenever there's food at work or when I get home."

When she was "on," Sandy's body was running on a steady diet of adrenaline, and it had no idea what to expect in terms of fuel. Sometimes Sandy gave her belly a feast of pizza, donuts,

3 celery stalks, diced
3 orange carrots, diced
1 large white onion, diced
5 tablespoons olive oil
3 teaspoons pink sea salt, divided
3 Yukon gold potatoes, chopped into cubes
1 orange pepper, diced

Sauté the celery, carrots, and onion with the olive oil and 1 teaspoon salt on medium heat for 10 minutes or until golden, while stirring.

Add 13 cups filtered water.

Add the potatoes, pepper, and remaining 2 teaspoons salt.

Bring to a boil, then turn the heat down to simmer for 30 minutes.

Let the soup cool for 1½ hours.

and wine in two-hour intervals, and sometimes it had to go ten hours between meals. When her adrenaline slowed down and there was no fuel source, Sandy crashed. Her body wondered where its massive, constant influx of food was and, when it didn't get it, it caused Sandy's physical and mental state to fluctuate wildly.

My goal was to introduce her to predictable eating times during a twenty-four-hour period so that she'd have a steady source of energy—not too much and not too little. So I returned to the notion of anchor times.

"Skip a solid food breakfast and drink liquids till lunch," I explained. "Then eat your first lunch around 12 or 1, your second at 3 or 4, and dinner at 7 or 8. You need to do this even when you're at work."

Sandy decided to set her phone's alarm for these anchor times. When her phone buzzed at noon, she could go to the break room and—deliberately and carefully—eat a portion of food she'd stashed in a container in the fridge. I coached her through how to find her zone, and when she hit it, she knew she could put the half-full container back. She could then take it out again at 3 or 4 for second lunch.

Within a week, Sandy was eating less and getting her energy back. Her trips to the gym energized her rather than exhausted her, and mornings on her day off became productive, not depressing. The lack of structure in Sandy's daily food intake was the biggest contributor to her lack of portion control, and the two issues were feeding off each other. The more often she grazed, the more she ate, and the more she ate, the more often she grazed.

Portion control will give you your power back. Food is pure energy, so when you give your body exactly what it needs at the times it needs it, it's going to power you through almost anything. Think of that campfire again. If you keep putting nice, dry logs that are not too big and not too small on it at regular intervals, it's going to burn steadily all through the night. Don't you want that kind of predictable, powerful energy all the way down to your cells?

5.

Eat Healthy Foods

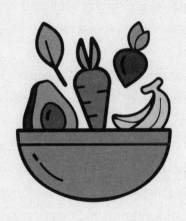

My son's preschool PTA hosts a small lecture series for the moms and dads. One night every few months, we meet at someone's house, settle into our chairs, and listen to authors, doctors, and other experts talk about everything from potty training to sleep to what to do about screen time. Last year, the committee asked me to speak, so, using my training as a culinary chef and certified health educator, I pulled together a presentation on making healthy meal choices for the family.

This PTA community, like most around the country, shares one common denominator. We want straight answers and solid direction so we can make the best possible decisions for our children. We're the kind of people who are up on the latest research, listen to all the experts, and are eager to throw our faith behind whatever is most scientifically sound and cutting edge. We've read books on developmental milestones, and we desperately want healthy, happy children and a well-balanced family.

The PTA hadn't given away any clues about what my take on food and family would be to other participants, so a few moms asked me beforehand what I might be talking about.

"I want you to be surprised," I answered, "but I think you're going to love it."

Knowing most people in the group, I was sure they were expecting hard-nosed advice. They were prepared for me to tell them to stop feeding their children sugar, to put their whole family on a gluten-free diet, or to cook reishi mushrooms with every dinner. Health advice from a can-do mom and health-based entrepreneur like me—who turned her life around by working extremely hard—is usually strict, right? Not all the time. When I got up in front of everyone and gave advice that was the exact opposite of strict, I think they were *shocked*.

"I'm not going to tell you what to buy and cook," I said. "What I am going to tell you is how to manage your time and your kitchen so you can make the best possible choices. This lecture is about time management; it is about being organized and creating a routine that allows you to eat healthy foods you enjoy. You know what's best for your family, so *you* are in charge."

That's right. You can choose, cook, and consume the healthiest, highest-quality foods simply by planning, getting organized, and never taking your decisions for granted. When you take control of your time and your kitchen, you position yourself in a positive structure that moves you—and your diet—forward with momentum. Eating as healthfully as possible may look different for each person, but the ways to make those choices are simple and universal.

Self-Awareness and Good Eating Habits

I'm a big fan of Gary Vaynerchuk (aka GaryVee). Gary is an entrepreneur, investor, public speaker, podcaster, and *New York Times* bestselling author who has established himself as an expert on entrepreneurship, marketing, and leadership. Gary came to this country from Belarus when he was three and started working at his dad's liquor store when he was fourteen. By the time he was twenty-seven, he'd built it from a small shop into an e-commerce site making $60 million a year.

One of the things I love most about watching and listening to GaryVee's posts (which I do all the time) is that he is so true to himself. He knows who he is and isn't ashamed of it, and he's made that self-awareness his motto. Gary constantly talks about his belief that you can't have happiness unless you know who you are. We all have weaknesses, he says, so we shouldn't try to deny them. Instead, we should realize what our strengths are and do everything we can to cultivate them. Gary worked with wine, loved wine, and knew that other people love it, too, so he made it his mission to put his family business on the internet and sell as much wine as he possibly could. If you have been building wooden chairs and tables since you were ten, and you derive more pleasure from it than anything else in life, you are probably meant to be a woodworker. Don't listen to your dad, who wants you to be a lawyer, because if you go to law school, you won't enjoy it because it's not your passion or purpose. Accept that you can make beautiful chairs, build your own business, and feel joy in what you do. Don't try to change that just because you're worried about earning lots of money or making your dad feel proud of you. Because if you try to mold yourself to someone else's image of you, you are never, ever going to feel passionate about your life.

I feel the same about the healthy foods you choose to eat. You are not like your thin best friend or the celebrity you see on the cover of a magazine. You are *you*, so own your choices. If you hate kale, do not make kale chips or kale salads and choke them down because you think they're good for you. If you love eggs, find as many healthy egg dishes as you can and incorporate them into your routine. And if you love carbs, do not be like my client Tara, who broke down crying in a session with me when I told her the diet she was on was probably not right for her.

"Thank you so much," she said. "I knew what I was eating wasn't making me happy."

Tara went on to explain that she and her husband had been trying to eat a protein-heavy diet because their best friends had lost weight following one. Plus, she'd read in a book that our ancestors didn't have access to carbs, so eating them wasn't a healthy or natural part of a good diet.

The problem was that she'd grown up in a big Italian family who loved to cook, and skipping her traditional Sunday pasta and meatball dinner made her miserable. In fact, her great joy in life was spending Sunday morning baking fresh bread and making homemade pasta for her family. Even though she'd put on fifteen pounds after having her second baby and she desperately wanted to lose it so she could get her energy back, she wasn't sure that letting go of the pasta-rich part of her life was worth it.

"Sunday dinner with just meatballs and no bread or pasta just feels *wrong*," she said.

It *was* wrong for Tara, and she was never going to be happy or make strides with her health if she cut grains out of her life. I suggested she limit her pasta intake to three servings during the work week, keeping her portions small enough that she didn't feel overstuffed. On Sundays, she could make her beloved homemade pasta and bread just like always. But she shouldn't eat until she felt sick to her stomach. Tara was open to that, and, as someone who listened to every podcast from every health expert, she was also delighted that it was backed up by research.

While I haven't put a name on my method of choosing healthy foods, doctors and scientists usually call it "intuitive eating." Intuitive eating promotes the idea that there is no such thing as a "good" or "bad" food, and that diets that lead people to eat foods they're not inclined to like (or that they actively dislike) will backfire. This is true; most people who follow restrictive diets initially lose weight, then gain it right back. More than that, they develop an unhealthy relationship with food. A 2008 survey conducted by the University of North Carolina at Chapel Hill looked at just over 4,000 American women and discovered that a full 75 percent of them struggle with some sort of disordered relationship with food, from anorexia to a desire to lose weight even though they are already at a healthy weight.

On the flip side, other studies revealed that when women decide to eat intuitively—choosing nutritious foods that they are naturally drawn to—they develop a better body image than those who restrict themselves. Intuitive eaters also stop bingeing on "bad" foods because they aren't forbidden anymore, and they move toward eating them in moderation and in combination with the healthier foods that they also love.

When I worked with private clients as a health educator, I found the concept of intuitive eating held true for almost all my clients. They hadn't merely shut down when they were told by diet experts or doctors not to eat certain foods; they actively sought out those foods. Think about when you were a child and your mom told you not to touch something she had put in the refrigerator. What did you do? You snuck up to the refrigerator while your mom was watching TV or in the bathroom and put your little fingers all over it. Foods that are "forbidden" are just too tempting to resist!

But when you take off any constraints, people embrace the freedom of choice and free will and make the food choices their hearts, minds, and stomachs tell them to make. They find their own way, and they discover how truly empowering that sense of ownership is. The reality is that people want to be the cause and not the effect. They want to follow their own instincts because empowerment feels *good*. It truly feels like progress is being made—and it is!

Take Tara. A few weeks after her tearful revelation about her new diet, she told me that once she'd started cooking pasta and bread on Sundays again, she hadn't craved carbs so much. She'd even begun eating them in sensible, healthy portions, trying gluten-free options, and experimenting with colorful salads and fresh vegetables that she could pair with her entrees. She looked forward to Sunday so much that she didn't want to spoil it by eating pasta on other days, and she decided to limit her pasta intake to two servings during the week (less than what I'd suggested). Her cravings lessened, and she lost five pounds in six weeks. Her

MOVE FORWARD EVERY DAY

You're probably thinking, *This is all great, MaryRuth, but what exactly am I supposed to eat? If I were left to my own devices to eat intuitively, I'd live on potato chips! I need direction. What do you consider a healthy meal?*

Like I said, only you understand what foods will make your body feel energized, strong, and satisfied, but know that a healthy meal is one that's fresh, unprocessed, and balanced. Shop at the perimeter of the grocery store where the less processed foods are kept—especially in the organic section of the produce aisle—and if you buy packaged products, choose those with as few ingredients as possible.

When you prepare a meal, remember that there are two types of food: nutrient-dense foods and water-dense foods. Nutrient-dense means that you get a significant amount of essential vitamins and nutrients (like protein) per calorie con-

powerful momentum had consistently built on itself, and the benefits were gradual, yet cumulative.

Getting Organized to Eat Healthy

I hear all the time from parents on social media how exhausting it is to plan and cook meals for their children. Back when many of these people were thinking about starting a family, they had

sumed without too many added sugars, fats, or sodium. Water-dense foods may also contain lots of nutrients, but they're offset by a high amount of water. Brown rice, beans, and animal protein are nutrient-dense; a salad or a serving of broccoli is water-dense. Root vegetables like beets and carrots don't have as much water, but they certainly contain more than meat or grains, so they fall into the water-dense category.

As you know, the body is made up mostly of water, and water-dense foods are an important source. But you can't ignore the nutrient-dense foods. My rule of thumb is that every meal should contain both. Pair salad with soba noodles or an egg frittata with vegetables. If you're indulging at lunch by ordering fish and chips, get a small salad, too. Don't forget to eat light to heavy, as we discussed on page 105, so eat the salad before the animal protein.

a vision that their children would be perfect eaters who would never beg for junk foods. These moms and dads would cook only "grown-up food," and their children would eat it up and ask for more.

Flash forward five years. These same people now have three children, and the oldest is allergic to eggs, milk, and peanut butter. The middle one *hates* anything green, and the youngest exists on a diet of toast with Nutella. The toast must be cooked for exactly one minute, thirty seconds, and if it's even slightly burned, they have to start from scratch. These moms and dads feel like they make breakfast, clean up, survive for the next three hours, make lunch, clean up, survive for the next three hours, then do the same at dinner, when there's an even bigger mess. They're terrified that their children are developing terrible eating habits, but they don't know what to do because the children don't like to eat *anything*. As far as meals are concerned, these moms' and dads' lives are constantly reactive; they ask, "What do you want for dinner?" at 6 p.m., rummage through the freezer, throw something on the stove, and then eat it in a hurry. Hours later, they collapse into bed, exhausted.

The body doesn't want to live reactively. That much adrenaline coursing through your veins keeps you going for a short time, but when it plummets, so do you.

Believe me, I know this feeling. My second son, Elliot, used to live on apples in the morning. If he didn't get one, he'd cry, bang his little fists on the tray of his highchair, and refuse to eat anything else. I tried so hard to calm him down that I was late starting my workday, and I had to ask my husband never to eat an apple before checking to see that there were others left.

Guys, it is *not worth it.* You deserve better than a rushed dinner of leftovers or an angry toddler hurling a banana through the air. You can avoid so much stress and heartache and ensure you're making the healthiest possible choices for your family—and living an efficient, energetic life—just by planning ahead *consistently* and *on a daily basis.* That's when you will see a big change in your life.

At 4 p.m. every day, most people's cortisol and blood-sugar levels start to plummet and they begin to think about how to wind down for the day. You're tired, slow, and not very reactive, so the thought of going to the grocery store on the way home from work, grabbing something healthy, then going home and cooking it, doesn't sound like such a good idea. You'd rather just order a pizza and eat it in front of the TV. In fact, when most of us don't have a plan for what to eat, we take the easy route and order takeout that's far less healthy than anything we might have cooked at home. Without a plan, we'll send our children to school with something prepackaged rather than something fresh.

Don't allow that to happen.

Here is my plan for you: before 4 p.m., you should always know what you're going to eat *the next day,* whether you'll need to go to the store, whether you might order takeout, if food will be served at your morning meeting, and, if you have children, what you might put in their lunchboxes. Writing it down on a Post-it can be helpful. Trust me, this planning will only take two minutes and it's life changing. You will never find yourself scrambling to figure out what to cook when you have three hungry teenagers sitting at the table. You will never wake up and realize you forgot to buy your toddler's beloved apples. You will never hear your stomach growl at a morning meeting because you thought there would be muffins there. While you plan for *tomorrow*, you can sit back and appreciate the fact that today is already taken care of.

WEEKLY MEAL PLAN

WEEK OF: _____

MONDAY
_____
_____
_____

TUESDAY
_____
_____
_____

WEDNESDAY
_____
_____
_____

THURSDAY
_____
_____

FRIDAY
_____
_____
_____

SATURDAY
_____
_____
_____

SUNDAY
_____
_____
_____

notes

If plotting out your meals one day in advance sounds restrictive, just remember: structure creates freedom. With your newfound freedom, you'll have more time and energy for things you enjoy, whether it's spending time with your partner or friends, working out, or taking a well-deserved rest after a hard day. Sure, you'll have to cook whatever you planned the day before, but it won't be stressful. You'll have your marching orders, so implementing them won't come as a shock. You'll feel empowered to think creatively about food, and you'll make healthy decisions because you won't be reactive. Adrenaline won't force you into hasty decisions; you'll know, for example, that you need to set aside five minutes to chop onions and peppers for a tomato sauce, so you won't rush to the grocery aisles looking for something you don't really love.

Taking Inventory Is Pure Discipline and So Worth It!

Unlocking the secret of healthy eating is as easy as opening your fridge once a day and taking a close look inside. Every morning, I wake up before my husband and children, wander down to the kitchen, take my vitamins, and make my celery juice. While I'm drinking it, I open up my refrigerator and take inventory. As the vitamins and juice energize my brain, I notice if I need more carrots, I pick up the coconut milk container and weigh whether I should buy more, and I look in the vegetable drawer, seeing what I could possibly cook the next day. I count how many apples and bananas are in the fruit bowl, and I open up the pantry, taking note of the fullness of the box of my son's favorite chickpea cereal. I look at expiration dates, counting ahead to see how many days I have before food goes bad. If there's any spoiled food, I dispose of it.

The whole time I'm doing this, I'll add items to my grocery list. Just by looking at what I have in my refrigerator and pantry, I can visualize what I might cook for my family throughout the week. Ideas I came up with the day before will change or grow. *I'll cook carrots since we have so many of them,* I may think. Or, *I think we need to cook vegetable soup Friday rather than tomorrow. We just had soup last night!*

Some people take kitchen inventory once a week, right before they go grocery shopping. I think this is overwhelming, so I don't recommend it. You'll forget to add things to your list. Or you'll discover rotten fruit buried in the fruit bowl and get mad at yourself. Your son might interrupt you, begging for a snack, and what you thought would take you twenty minutes will take you half an hour. Then you'll be late to soccer practice. Instead, take five minutes once a day, at whatever time is best for you, and I promise you'll not only start to choose healthier foods, but you'll feel on top of your life.

Research supports the idea that an organized home leads you to make decisions that are better for your body. Three different experiments published together in 2013 looked at two groups of people: one whose homes were disorderly and one whose homes were tidy. When asked to choose between an apple or a piece of chocolate for a snack, the people who surrounded themselves with order rather than chaos were two times more likely to choose the apple. Organization isn't just good for your home; it's good for *you*!

I had a client named Eric who grew up in a working-class family in a small apartment in New York City. His parents were huge partiers who'd met at a club in their early twenties, then dated casually for a few months. When Eric's mom got pregnant, they'd been shocked. A baby was the *last* thing they wanted or needed. But they decided to try to make it work, so they got married and had Eric, then they had his brother two years later. Raising two children before you're ready is a tough position to find yourself in, and Eric's mom spent their childhood looking for an escape. She would sneak out a few nights a week to drink with her friends, then return home and fight with Eric's dad. When Eric was ten, his dad announced he'd had enough and filed for divorce. Eric could count on two hands the times he saw his father after that.

Eric's mom had never had a steady job, but she needed money badly, so she scrambled and got work that paid minimum wage. Her hours were all over the place, so Eric and his brother fended for themselves, doing their homework alone, and living on the chips, sugary cereal, and cans of soda that were lying around the kitchen. Eric's mom still loved to party, so when she was home her friends came over and drank all night while Eric tried to sleep. He'd wake up in the morning and discover there was no food in the refrigerator, so he'd go to school hungry, hating that his life was never, ever in control.

Eric was a smart guy, and he graduated at the top of his high school class, got a scholarship to a good college, and became an

MOVE FORWARD EVERY DAY

Knowing what food you have on hand can be helpful at the most unexpected times. How many times have you gotten an email from your child's class parent or teacher asking you to bring a dessert or a fruit salad to a class party at the end of the week? Or what about that potluck supper your friend decided to throw that you completely forgot about? Have you dreaded the idea of making something, thinking, *Great. Now I have to dream up a recipe and go to the store some night after work.* If you already knew what you had on hand and had stocked up weeks before on those occasionally-used-but-not-vital items like chocolate chips and cassava flour, or easy-to-freeze entrees like quiche or soup, you'd already have everything you need. No grocery store trips necessary! You'll show up looking uber prepared, when in actuality all you did was stay on top of the food you have on hand.

accountant at a big Manhattan firm. He made a good living, but he couldn't shake the feeling that poverty and hunger were one lost paycheck away. He carried about forty extra pounds because food meant comfort and security, and he practically lived on frozen dinners, chips, and Chinese takeout because he'd never learned to cook. His refrigerator was also a mess because he couldn't stand the thought of wasting food. Even if the ketchup in his refrigerator was five years old, he would *not* throw it away.

Eric came to me at the recommendation of someone in his office after he'd told her he wanted to lose weight. But right away I learned there was more to his agenda.

"Growing up, we never had enough food, and I just don't know how to eat well. I want to be able to buy things that are healthy, will last a long time, and will give me some bang for my buck. I just want to feel in control of what's in my house because I never felt that way growing up."

The first thing I talked to Eric about was organizing his kitchen. When he looked horrified at my suggestion that he weed out some of the chips and cookies in his pantry and donate them to a food bank, I realized his food issues were about much more than his fear of going hungry. Eric had grown up in a house with no discipline, and he'd been unable to create healthy boundaries between himself and what he ate because of that.

I recently ran across a quote from the actor Will Smith, which summed up everything I feel about discipline. "Discipline is the strongest form of self-love," Smith wrote. "It is ignoring current pleasures for bigger rewards to come. It's loving yourself enough to give you everything you've ever wanted."

Neither of Eric's parents had had the discipline to be real care-takers, and they always acted on impulse, thinking of short-term gains rather than the long-term good. Everything had been fleeting with them: marriage, jobs, children, and nights out. Eric had never felt true ownership of anything; all the junk food he stocked in his kitchen could slip through his fingers at a moment's notice, so he held on to it for dear life. I wanted to teach him how to account for and place importance on the value of food—which, in turn, would allow him to care for himself.

"Discipline involves looking at the big picture," I told him. "For you, the big picture is cleaning out your kitchen so you can clean out your body. By being disciplined enough to wake up a little earlier and go through your refrigerator, you can take inventory of what is really good for you."

My hope was that Eric could begin to see himself not as the poor boy with the dysfunctional mom, but as a successful individual who didn't need to keep bad food around. Throwing away or donating a few frozen dinners didn't mean he was wasting anything; it just meant he loved himself enough to know he deserved better than junk food. When he realized what it was that he *truly* needed, he could start making healthy food choices and move forward in his life.

Every Action Counts

So much power comes from the small actions you make in your life, so I'm urging you never, ever to take them for granted or disregard them. Think of Eric; if he hadn't taken that small step of looking through his refrigerator and pantry every day, he wouldn't have started feeling more confident when he went to the grocery store. That confidence led him to buy vegetables and fresh items he'd heard of but never tried, which led him to start cooking. As he cooked healthier foods, he began to lose weight—a lot of it. Soon, he felt comfortable registering for an online dating site. After a few months of bad first dates, he met someone who just happened to have grown up in his neighborhood, and they got engaged within a year.

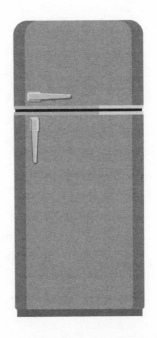

Every object, person, action, and reaction in the world is composed of energy. Especially in families, if there is one person who's a weak link, casting negative energy, everyone else is affected. Look at Eric's family; the disorder was contagious. Think about that Thanksgiving when your aunt and uncle were fighting, and your aunt was so upset she burned the apple pie and undercooked the turkey. That negative energy had repercussions for *everyone*. A moldy, rotten piece of food sitting in your refrigerator has stagnant, negative energy, too. It's signaling that you're ignoring aspects of good health, wasting money, and not paying attention to the healthy items you could be cooking for your family. But if you're spending five focused minutes every morning taking inventory of the foods in your house, you'll have five extra minutes at night to watch your favorite show rather than scrambling to figure out what to cook for dinner.

You might laugh, but I swear that not letting any food in my refrigerator go bad is one of the major reasons my mom and I got out of debt. Just by knowing exactly what I had—and cooking it or packing it away for lunch—I never overspent at the store or ordered overpriced takeout. I was like a restaurant owner who understood that my business had a razor-thin profit margin, and one forgotten or bad piece of food was money lost. I estimate I saved at least a hundred dollars a month from what I'd spent before on food. My micro action connected to the macro, and I was able to move my life forward in a fundamentally positive way, toward a life free of crippling money problems. Because of

MOVE FORWARD EVERY DAY

For over twelve years I've had a green juice every day. From beets to celery to kale to cucumbers, if you can juice it, I've tried it. But by far, the best juice and juicing regime I've ever done is drinking one sixteen-ounce glass of celery juice every morning on an empty stomach.

I *love* celery juice for all its dozens of health benefits. It is rich in vitamins K, A, B2, B6, and C, plus the nutrients folate, potassium, manganese, and pantothenic acid. It has loads of phytonutrients with anti-inflammatory and antioxidant properties, and it helps lower cholesterol, fight allergies, aid digestion, lower blood pressure, fight infections, boost immunity, and improve cardiovascular health. It restores hydrochloric acid

this consistent hard work, today my family and I enjoy financial stability.

Remember how you felt during those first few uncertain, confusing, and overwhelming weeks when COVID-19 began to ravage the communities around us. If your impulse was to drink a bottle of wine or eat a pan of brownies, you're definitely not alone, but you knew that would make the following day feel like a year. If you made a small action like drinking a green juice, cleaning out your refrigerator, or ordering healthy foods for delivery, I'm sure it had a *huge* impact. Your family ate better. Your body felt energized. Your kitchen wasn't a mess that made you feel frustrated.

in the gut, helps the liver flush out fat and toxins, and some studies even show that it improves fertility!

Every morning, I take one bunch of celery, wash it carefully, and cut off the stalks. Celery is high on the list of foods that pesticides most affect, so I always choose organic celery. Then I place it in my juicer and, *voila*, I have sixteen ounces of juice. I usually add stevia because I think it improves the taste, but you don't have to. Just drink your juice straight out of a glass because if you use a straw the digestive enzymes in your mouth won't touch the juice, which is key to absorbing all its wonderful nutrients. Swish the juice around in your mouth, too, to fully cover it with enzymes.

These small actions moved you forward in subtle, powerful ways during one of the toughest times our society has ever known. You didn't have to run a marathon or get a promotion to feel good; all it took was one small, simple action full of good energy that snowballed into healthy momentum. No matter how hard the challenges were in front of you—or still are—you can overcome them one small action at a time. Why not start by reorienting and reorganizing your life so that you eat healthy foods? Don't take that simple decision for granted. It counts and, together with the other actions, it will add up to big gains. One day, you will know this to be true in the core of your heart.

6.

Get Fifteen Minutes of Direct Sunshine Each Day

Vitamin D is crucial for the mind and body!

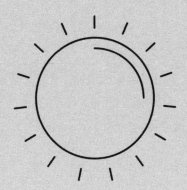

Unless your house is tucked inside a canyon, it's hard not to find a sunny spot in Los Angeles. Where I live is no exception. Nearly every side of my house gets a blast of light between sunrise to sunset, and it pours into the windows that line the top and bottom floors. But there's one side that always gets a little sunnier, and that's where my son Ethan's bathroom is.

I love houseplants, so I put a small one on the windowsill in there, hoping that one day Ethan would water and care for it without my help. It's just a simple green plant that loves a hot, dry place like LA. This little plant started with four buds that were each about an inch long and reached in different directions, like a four-leaf clover. Two years later, those sprouts are now giant tentacles that have climbed up and out of the pot. They don't spread apart anymore but instead lean toward the window, seeking the sun that streams in throughout the day. The arms of the plant are firm and strong, soaking in every delicious drop of sunshine they can get.

I look at that little plant all the time when I'm giving Ethan a bath, and I think about what it takes for it to thrive. Just like every plant, its needs are simple: water, nutrient-rich soil, clean air, and sunshine, which allows it to sprout, blossom, and grow. The light energy from the sun is that plant's main food source, and when the chlorophyll-containing proteins in its cells absorb the sun's rays, they convert it into chemical energy that powers every single one of its processes. Without sun, the plant begins to starve, and it turns in on itself as it wilts, withers, and eventually dies.

Humans aren't that much different from plants. Sure, on a cellular level, we can survive without sun, and there are entire communities of people who live near the poles and spend months of the year huddled inside, then watch the sun peek over the horizon for only a few hours a day. But when the sun climbs higher and stays there longer, they rush outside, stretching their bodies toward the light.

I once had a client who came to see me right after she'd come back from a business trip to Sweden. She arrived in Stockholm about a week before the summer solstice, when the sun rises around 4 a.m., hangs above eye level and moves slowly across the sky all day, then starts to dip around 9 p.m. When my client stepped out of the cab that took her from the airport to her hotel, she looked up and saw a small park lined with folding chairs.

"It was wonderful, MaryRuth," she said. "The whole park was full of people sitting in chairs, and they were all turned toward the sun with their heads raised up, their eyes closed, and their faces bathed in light."

After a long, dark winter and short spring, each of those people were just like Ethan's plant. They sat soaking in the sun and gathering up energy that gave them strength, healed them on the cellular level, and put them in a mindset that would move them forward every day. I firmly believe a minimum of fifteen minutes in the sun—without your sunglasses on, which I will explain later—is a tiny, effortless, universal action that grows and multiplies, powering you through tough times or allowing you to take a good situation to the next level. While it might seem insignificant—something you can skip or take for granted—it's also a powerful reminder of all that's good. Most people feel much happier and more energized after sitting in the sun for fifteen minutes.

The Power of Cellular Intelligence

We all make mistakes. Sometimes, they're silly and small, like when you accidentally knock a glass jar to the ground while you're reaching into the pantry for a box of cereal. Other times, they're deliberate and just plain wrong, like when you cheat on your high school calculus test and get caught. Those are the times when small errors in judgment become massive mess-ups with consequences that are *huge*.

This was the case with Maria, one of the most inspiring clients I ever had. Maria had been a junior at a college in Upstate New York about ten years before I first met her. She was an average student who never failed any of her classes, but she definitely liked the social side of college more than studying. One night a few months after her twenty-first birthday, Maria and her roommates decided to go to a party at a house a few miles off campus.

Maria was supposed to be the designated driver, but when she walked into the party, she was suddenly terrified by the thought that everyone there was having more fun than she was. If she wasn't drinking, would she even fit in? As the music started blasting, Maria spied a guy across the room she'd been interested in for months and she worried that without a drink she'd never be able to talk to him. So she grabbed a shot of vodka and knocked it back. A few minutes later, she reached for a beer and her confidence started to grow.

Around midnight—four hours after they'd arrived at the party—Maria's friends walked over to her and announced that they wanted leave. Maria was three beers and two shots in, but she thought to herself, *Whatever. I've always been a good driver, and it's straight all the way home.* She and her friends stumbled out of the party. Then she dug her keys out of her purse and settled in behind the wheel as she started up the car. She put her foot on the gas, drove down the driveway, and pulled out into the road. That's the last thing she remembered.

When Maria woke up in the hospital two days later, she couldn't feel her legs.

"I'm so sorry, baby," her mom said, stroking her hair, "but you're paralyzed from the waist down."

The man who'd broadsided her at 40 mph was the only one who could recall Maria driving her car into oncoming traffic. By some miracle, the driver had escaped with only a concussion and a few broken ribs, and Maria's friends had walked away with cuts and bruises. But Maria's life would never be the same.

"I spent five weeks in the hospital and two months in rehab," she said.

I've never suffered a physical injury like Maria, so I can't fully understand what she endures. But I do know from the hours we spent together that Maria's broken body and mind were similar to what I went through mentally when my dad and brother passed away suddenly. Even though she was in pain, her cells were strong and smart, and they wanted to fight toward health. Just like the little plant in Ethan's window, her body was going to put in every effort to grow toward what was going to restore it.

Our bodies have a deeply ingrained cellular intelligence. When a virus invades a cell, it creates antibodies that will recognize and fight that same strain of virus if it comes back. This amazing memory is reinforced by repetition, and the more often these efficient little machines act on autopilot, the stronger they become. Cells thrive on a consistent diet of high-quality foods and a good amount of sleep at regular intervals and, over time, they grow used to them. If something sets them back—like an injury, illness, or addiction—they may suffer, but they can find their groove again and start to mend. They know exactly what they need to do to restore themselves. Just think of what happens to a plant that's kept away from light or not given enough water; as soon as it's given the proper nutrition, it perks right back up.

What I find so encouraging is that we have some control over our cellular intelligence. Regularly and consistently giving your body the good energy it needs is within your power—and best of all, it can be so simple. What's one of the things you can do? Just get out into the sun without sunglasses for fifteen minutes a day, and let the gorgeous rays bathe your face.

"When I found out I was paralyzed," said Maria, "it would have been so easy to tell my body it was time to give up. I could have stayed in bed and refused to do physical therapy or anything good for myself. But I know my body doesn't want that. It wants to repair itself, but it relies on me to give it the right tools."

Maria's medical team knew this, too, so as soon as she was safely able to leave her bed, the nurses lifted her up and placed her in a wheelchair, then took her outside. As she soaked in the sun's rays, her cells tapped into their memory bank, focusing on their natural inclination to heal.

How Sunshine Heals

Letting the sun wash over your face doesn't just feel good. It's also a pure dose of good energy for every part of your being. Let's break down how this works.

The sun emits electromagnetic rays in the form of visible light, ultraviolet light, infrared, radio waves, x-rays, and gamma rays. While some of these are harmful—like ultraviolet light (UV), which damages your DNA and can lead to skin cancer—others are good for you.

For example, when red and near-infrared light (on the visible and invisible ends of the spectrum, respectively) penetrate the layers of your skin, they cause your mitochondria—the so-called power centers of your cells—to make more energy. An increase in energy then speeds up the body's healing mechanisms, especially because it helps tissue grow and reduces inflammation. Red and near-infrared light are now used to treat certain types of cancer, dementia, dental pain, wounds, dermatological scars, sun damage, and visible signs of aging.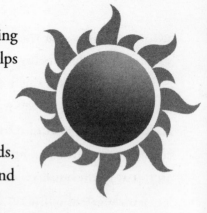

Exposing your skin to sunlight also triggers a photosynthetic reaction in your cells that leads to the production of vitamin D. While you can get a daily dose of vitamin D from fish, eggs, and supplements, this essential vitamin is much more abundant in sunlight. It's estimated that half of Americans don't get enough vitamin D, which is terrible news because vitamin D helps improve bone health and brain function, dramatically decreases the risk of autoimmune diseases like type 1 diabetes and multiple sclerosis, and helps prevent osteoporosis. In the right doses, vitamin D also reduces the risk of cancer—particularly breast cancer, whose risk can decline by as much as 80 percent!

Research also shows that sunlight helps boost your body's immunity. Michael D. Hollick, a professor of medicine at Boston University, published a study that showed that vitamin D increases the expression of hundreds of genes that regulate immune function, therefore helping us better fight infections. And a 2016 study from the Georgetown University Medical Center discovered that when the immune system's T cells are exposed to low levels of the blue light that's found in the sun's visible spectrum, they increase their responsiveness to harmful pathogens and cancer cells.

Using the sun to help speed healing wasn't the smart idea of a few modern scientists and Maria's doctors. It has been an integral part of hospital protocols for over a hundred years. Florence Nightingale advocated so hard for patients to get sun that many early twentieth-century hospitals were built with skylights and large east-facing windows. And, during the 1918–1919 flu pandemic, people who were housed in outdoor overflow tents and exposed to the sun died at far lower rates than those who stayed inside.

You might be wondering, *If getting sun on my skin is what's so good for me, why do you recommend I take off my sunglasses?* Because letting the sun wash over your skin is only half the story. Within your retinas—the layer of tissue that lines the back of your eyes—exist photoreceptor cells that absorb light. When they sense light, these cells send signals through the optic nerve to the small part of the brain called the *hypothalamus*. Among other things, the hypothalamus controls the body's circadian rhythm, or the mechanism by which you regulate your internal functions. When your eyes receive as little as fifteen minutes of bright light, it resets your body's circadian rhythms, signaling that you should be awake. Just remember that you should never look directly at the sun because doing so could cause permanent damage to your eyes.

People who work the night shift or spend too much time indoors in front of a screen—which, let's be honest, is *many* of us—often don't receive this healing fifteen-minute shot of sunshine during the day. Not being exposed to the sun long enough—or at all—throws off our circadian rhythm, which then affects our metabolism. An off-kilter metabolism can cause a bunch of additional issues, including digestive problems, low energy, and decreased immunity. Research also shows that people who work at night tend to be heavier than those who are out and about during the day. But let's focus on the positive, because the solution is simple, free, and accessible to everyone. Just get out into the sun once during the day for fifteen minutes, and you can help avoid or reverse all these issues.

Getting fifteen minutes of sunshine is also proven to help you fall asleep at night. The hormone melatonin, which regulates the sleep–wake cycle, is produced by the brain's pineal gland when the retina senses light and sends a signal through the optic nerve. During the morning—when light levels are high—melatonin production declines and we wake up. At night, it increases and helps us fall asleep. Research shows, however, that people who work at night produce lower levels of melatonin. This happens because these workers are exposed to light during the evening, which suppresses the body's natural production of this essential hormone. So, it follows that if you want to sleep at night, you should give your body plenty of daytime light and turn the lights off when it's time for bed.

The effects of a good night's sleep are immediate, including mood improvement. But sleep isn't the only key to a general sense of well-being. The hormone serotonin, which your brain produces

MOVE FORWARD EVERY DAY

There are two types of sunscreen. The first is mineral sunscreen, whose main ingredients are usually zinc oxide or titanium dioxide. Mineral sunscreen literally lies on the skin and acts as a barrier against UV rays. Chemical sunscreens, on the other hand, contain synthetic ingredients that work by penetrating the layers of the skin, then absorbing the sun's harmful rays and releasing them as heat.

I strongly recommend only using mineral sunscreen because it's nontoxic. When you wear chemical sunscreen and the sun opens up your pores, the toxic chemicals enter your bloodstream at levels up to 438 times the recommended amounts. These ingredients can create hormonal disruptions, enter breast milk that can then pass to a baby, and can still be found on the skin and in the blood weeks later. Some toxic sunscreens are also responsible for neurological issues in babies and young children, and many of them are contributing to the destruction of ocean life and coral reefs. So, skip the scary chemicals and always choose a nontoxic sunscreen, which is far safer and just as effective.

more of when it senses the sun, also controls your mood. When levels are high, you may be happy and calm, and when they're low, you're likely anxious and depressed. But before you pack your bags and move to Florida thinking that a warm, sunny place is the key to a lifetime of happiness, know that weather doesn't affect serotonin production. Any amount of sun at any time of year will increase the levels of serotonin in your brain. All you have to do is get outside and take off your sunglasses for fifteen minutes.

Researchers estimate that the light exposure we get from being outside is a thousand times more powerful than what we receive inside, so I can't stress enough that opening the shades and letting the sun stream in isn't enough. Your windows are likely filtering out many of the sun's healing rays. If you're too sick to get up and out, open a window and get as close to it as you can. Or if you're insanely busy at work for twelve hours a day, just sneak outside for fifteen minutes to grab lunch. The key is to do the best you possibly can. I don't expect you to be perfect, but you can make progress, and those baby steps forward may make all the difference in your energy levels, your mood, your sleep, and your immune system.

Being Present

For many of you, meditation is hugely powerful. Whether you're sitting in silence first thing in the morning, clearing your thoughts and focusing on your breath, or whether you're silently repeating a mantra to yourself, this practice has changed many lives.

For some of you, though, meditation may not feel right. That's completely normal! Meditation is not for everyone. I am sure the problem isn't that you're avoiding the peace that comes with learning to be present. Perhaps meditation feels too forced or doesn't fit in your routine when you just want to get your day going and start your to-do list. I also know there are a lot of you out there who may leave a short practice feeling frustrated or incompetent because it doesn't seem like anything has changed inside you. You're still anxious, depressed, lethargic, unmotivated, or lacking any sense of inner peace. While it's true that the benefits of meditation usually take time, you may just need to find another way to quiet your mind.

How about trying something that's simple, free, and available to everyone? Step outside and soak in the sun for fifteen minutes. This can be your form of meditation.

The benefits of being present cannot be overstated. Not only does research show that, over time, it reduces depression, pain, and anxiety, and increases brain processing, focus, and emotional regulation, it also just feels good in the moment. Think of this: The receptive, sensory portion of your brain is like the surface of the ocean, always moving and reacting to every stimulus that comes its way. When you dive down, though, there's a natural silence. Deep in the folds of your mind—just like in the bottom of the ocean—you can find pure, lasting calm. Your natural tendency is to seek that quiet. When you allow yourself to surrender to the fact that life is what it is—even for just fifteen minutes—you unburden yourself of the reactive part of your brain that seeks to control everything. You stop overthinking what you should have done in the past or should do in the future, and you accept what is.

In the early days of her hospitalization, when Maria sat outside in the sun for fifteen minutes, she told me she still felt sad and angry. Sometimes she hated herself for how careless she'd been, and much of the time she worried about how she was going to live a life that had been so dramatically changed.

"But, just sitting there, soaking up all that energy, I knew, at that moment, there was nothing I had to do. For fifteen minutes, I could just let life *be*."

Being present is a little bit different than being mindful. I think of being present as a state of focus in every moment. Mindfulness is broader; it involves acknowledging all the sensations associated with the present, then refusing to judge or dissect those feelings. Like Maria said, being present is allowing yourself to just exist. It's giving yourself the freedom not to dwell on the mistakes of the past or worry about the future. Being present is a feeling; it's that focused, Eye of the Tiger sensation when your senses are sharp and your energy is fluid. You feel almost as if you're unfolding and blossoming; you're open and vulnerable, capable of accepting the fact that you have no idea what the future will offer, but, for just a few minutes, you don't have to think about it.

Of course, you can't be fully present 100 percent of the time. You still need to take inventory of your refrigerator and think about what you might cook or eat the next day. No matter what, you still have to look at the calendar, plan your week, and question whether you can really handle going out two nights in a row or if your daughter can juggle three birthday parties on a Saturday. But for just a fraction of your long, busy day, you can sit in the sun and let your worries fall away while your mind enters a state of peace and quiet.

Know that—especially for you overachievers or adrenaline junkies—learning to be present can be *hard* work, but it's an essential part of the process of moving forward. Every time you relax and take a break, tell yourself that you are not being lazy or stagnant. You are rewarding yourself and doing something positive at the same time. And you're helping your immune system! Being present is a gift to you. It's a time to fill yourself with the good energy of the sun and the satisfaction that there is nothing the world is asking of you for just a little bit.

Energy Balance

At eighty years old, James was the oldest person I had ever worked with. He had led an incredibly active life, golfing three times a week, attending shows with his wife, and going out to dinner with friends as often as possible. Tall, strongly built, and not a pound overweight, he'd worked as a contractor until he was seventy-five and had quit only so he could take care of his wife after she received a diagnosis of breast cancer. Unfortunately, she didn't make it, and James had been a widower for about three years.

I could tell right away James was incredibly lonely. He talked more than most of my clients, eagerly making eye contact and asking if it was rude to text me every day to check in. He mentioned more than once that, while he had children and grand-children scattered around the country, he wished he felt up to traveling because phone and email just weren't enough. He also told me that when his wife passed away, he thought about start-ing up his business again, but decided it was too hard for an old man to compete with all the young contractors in New York.

"Besides," he said, "I'm so tired all the time now. I'm afraid I'd fall asleep on the job."

James said he'd started taking naps at least twice a day, and while he knew that wasn't unusual for a person in their eighties, he thought it was a bad sign that he woke up feeling just as tired as he'd been when he fell asleep. He enjoyed taking walks twice a day with his wife when she was alive, but now he was lucky if he got out once every two days. And golf? It was a distant memory.

"All my friends have moved to Florida or have died," he said, "so I haven't golfed in three years."

I always encourage my clients to get bloodwork done to deter-mine if any underlying conditions are causing their problems. While I'm not a doctor, I sensed just by looking at strong, fit James that he probably had nothing seriously wrong with him. He might suffer the fatigue, aches, and pains that so many older people do, but something told me that he probably just needed more stimulation in his life.

His blood test results proved it.

"James," I said, pushing his bloodwork toward him, "you are in better health than 99 percent of people in their eighties. That's fantastic news. So, you need to do everything you can to improve on the good health you already enjoy. Part of that involves increasing your vitamin D3 levels."

Once again, I pulled out a piece of paper from my desk and used a pencil to draw a big circle on it. This time, instead of dividing it into one-hour segments like I did with so many other clients, I moved my pencil around the circumference.

"James, you are at the center of this circle. You have energy inside and all around you, flowing continuously and in balance. Now, if I push too hard, this pencil lead will snap right off, or I'll rip the paper. Right?" He nodded. "But if I don't push hard enough, you can hardly see the circle. One swipe with an eraser and it's gone." I paused and put the pencil down. "Do you feel like your circle of energy is weak or strong?"

"No question," James answered, "it's weak."

"It's time to get it back in balance," I answered. "You'll know that all is well in your life when your internal energy matches your external energy."

James was healthy, strong, and eager to be active, with an internal fire burning inside him. But without a spouse, dinner dates, exercise, or even a regular practice of going outside, he had no external excitement. He was radiating more energy than he was receiving, and it was burning him out and leaving him exhausted.

Think about this: Have you ever *really* put your neck on the line? Maybe you tried hard to get someone to love you as much as you loved them, or maybe you worked hours of overtime at a job, hoping like crazy that you'd be rewarded with a promotion. In both those situations, you spent precious energy with the expectation that you'd get something back. When I decided to become a health educator, I paid money I didn't have on an advertisement for my services, then held my breath and crossed my fingers that it would work out. Luckily, it did, and I received as much energy as I gave. But if I'd been that person who loved and loved and then got dumped, or worked and worked and didn't get a raise, my internal energy wouldn't match my external energy. And I'd be exhausted, angry, or disappointed because of it.

MOVE FORWARD EVERY DAY

Everyone knows that too much screen time isn't good for you, but this is especially true at night. Computers, tablets, TVs, and phones emit short-wavelength blue light, which delays the release of sleep-inducing melatonin, increases alertness, and disrupts the body's circadian rhythms, effectively tricking the body into believing it's still daytime. Too much screen time is also associated with an increased risk for obesity, heart disease, cancer, and diabetes.

These issues are part of the reason researchers have again and again promoted the idea that we should turn off all screens one to two hours before bedtime. But if you just can't bear the thought of not bingeing on Netflix or checking your email before bed, there are other ways you can combat blue light:

EVERYDAY WELLNESS | 153

We depend on the world to give back as much as we give it, but the issue is that the external is out of our control. Spouses pass away. It rains on your wedding day. Or, on the positive side, you might sign up to run a half marathon and worry, *Am I up for this kind of challenge?* Your internal energy has to match your external energy, or you might not be able to move forward. On a daily basis, what you feel on the inside should match and be expressed to the outer world.

- This one's my favorite: a recent and very promising study out of Sweden showed that people who get plenty of daytime light don't experience any nasty blue light disruptions at night, even when they look at a screen right before going to bed. So, go outside and soak in the sun as much as you can!

- Amber-colored lenses, which are sold without a prescription, can block the absorption of blue light. Studies show that people who wear them and look at a screen at night don't experience a delayed release of melatonin.

- Some computer programs have been designed to adjust the light emission on your computer at night from blue light to a more sleep-friendly orange light. Just search for and download the one you like best.

Why not depend on the most consistent source of energy in the galaxy to help fire up your internal self? Sitting in the sun sounds like an insignificant thing, but it's a small action that can shift entire force fields of energy. Sure, there could be clouds in the sky, but even on a gray day in the dead of winter 80 percent of the sun's rays still come through. Going outside for fifteen minutes a day is a deliberate, dependable way to balance your internal and external energy, and it's exactly what I suggested to James he do.

I got a text from James a month or so after we first met.

Guess what, MaryRuth? I'm fostering a dog. We go to the dog park for an hour a day in the sunshine.

I kept up with James for the next year, and he told me not only had he decided to adopt the dog—it was a senior just like him—but he'd met a widow at the park. She liked to golf, so they'd started going every Saturday. He was down to one nap every other day and felt better than he had in years.

Sunshine is exceptionally powerful and healing. In the most painful days of each of my pregnancies—when I was throwing up all the time—I forced myself to go outside and sit in a lawn chair for at least fifteen minutes. I didn't bring my phone and I didn't wear my sunglasses. Instead, I thought about positive things, and my breath evened out, my stomach settled, and my mind woke up. My internal world might have been in despair from the bone-breaking nausea, but for those few minutes, my external world was at peace. As the sun beat down on me, it began to create an energetic harmony within my body. I didn't have to do anything, and just by being still, I moved forward.

MOVE FORWARD EVERY DAY

Whether or not you engage in a deliberate practice of meditation, or if you, like me, just prefer to sit in the sun once a day, using visualization can be incredibly helpful to slow down your mind. It can also improve your performance level. A study from Loyola Marymount University showed that dancers improve their jumping height by visualizing "the whole body is a spring." Michael Phelps, the Olympic gold medalist swimmer, has said in an interview that he uses visualization before big swim meets, too. Whether or not you have a goal in mind, here are some things you might like to visualize:

- Your body bathed in whatever color you find most relaxing and restorative.

- Lying on a float in the middle of a pool in the tropics.

- Your breath. Visualize your chest or belly rising and falling as your breath enters and leaves your body.

7.

Sleep Seven to Eight Hours

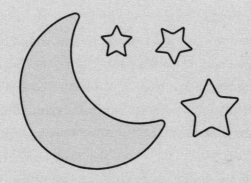

I magine that you spend a third of your life in water. Maybe you find yourself in a swimming pool where the water is the perfect temperature, and you have your choice of rafts or noodles to help you float. Or you might be in a mountain lake where you can swim to a dock if you need a break. Wherever you are, the swimming is fun, but it isn't always easy. Sometimes the water is choppy and other times you can't touch the bottom. For the eight hours a day you spend in the water, you'd want to be prepared, right? You'd be wearing the highest-quality wet suit and be covered in nontoxic sunscreen. You would have trained so much that you could probably qualify for the Olympics. There's no way you'd fly by the seat of your pants and get in the water *for a third of your life* without being diligent, strict, and on top of your game. For sure, you'd be the best swimmer you could possibly be.

Why don't we treat sleep the same way? Think about it. If you live to be seventy-five, you will spend a full twenty-five years either asleep or attempting to fall asleep. Sleep may feel like a passive pursuit, but it's actually a vigorous activity for your body and mind. More than that, it's the life jacket that allows you to sink or swim, and the foundation that gives you the strength and energy to take action to move forward every day. Yet too many people shrug off sleep as an afterthought or a bother, believing that there are a thousand more important things to do than to get in bed. I want to make it clear that you *cannot be casual about your sleep habits.* If you want to improve your life incrementally, starting within a twenty-four-hour period, you have to gain mastery of your sleep routine. Embracing this powerful state can change everything about your life, and gaining control of it can be straightforward if you take the right approach.

The Power of Chronological Order

When I first met Alex, he was a thirty-one-year-old PhD student in the computer science department of one of the top universities in New York City. His parents ran a convenience store in Queens, and they'd told him when he was in third grade that paying for college was going to be a struggle for them. Alex didn't resent his parents because of this—he knew they were doing their very best in a really tough line of work—but he decided that, money or not, he was going to go to a great college. He studied like crazy, never missed a day of school, and graduated second in his high school class. He got a scholarship to a fantastic university, worked in a lab when he wasn't in the library, and graduated summa cum laude with honors. A few years after starting his career at a major tech company, he decided that the best way to advance there—or anywhere—was to go back to school. His company saw his potential and agreed to pay for most of his tuition. Alex landed in a PhD program, absolutely thrilled to be back in school.

Alex came to me at the advice of one of his advisors, who'd been my client the year before.

"I'm worried about him," he told me in a text. "Don't tell him I told you this, but he's just not the same ambitious guy he was last year."

Alex trudged into my office on 47th and Third, then slumped back in a chair and folded his arms. He wasn't overweight and he didn't look out of shape, but he seemed distracted, focusing more on what was on my wall than the fact I was about to ask him a question.

"How are you feeling?" I asked.

"Oh, I'm okay," he answered, "but I just don't have the energy I used to have. I'm falling asleep in class and not able to work as late at night as I usually do. I'm on a huge research project now, and I just can't risk messing up on it. But I worry I will if I can't focus better."

The more Alex and I talked about his eating habits and his exercise routine, the more I wondered how he could have such low energy. To save money, he'd moved back in with his mom and dad, but he still made time to go to the gym a few times a week. He ate healthy food, took the family dog for a walk every morning, and had a positive attitude about life. He was grateful for his family and education and was eager to work his way up in a career that would make his parents proud and give them more stability. But by Alex's own words, something was missing.

"I have all of these positive things in my life," he said. "For some reason, though, I can't really enjoy them."

I already had a piece of paper and pen on my desk, so I drew a circle on it as Alex scooted his chair toward me. I divided the circle into twelve hour-long chunks and circled three anchor times: 12–1 p.m., 3–4 p.m., and 7–8 p.m. Then I moved my pencil up toward 10 p.m. and marked it with an X.

"Alex," I said, "we're going to come back to this schedule I'm about to propose to you. First, however, I want to make one thing clear. I believe everyone going into my program has to approach it in four successive phases. The order you go about tackling your health is very important, and if you don't act on your first intention, there's no way you're going to have the energy or motivation to accomplish your second."

That's when I introduced Alex to my notion of chronological order.

Before you embark on a major change in your life that will allow you to move forward out of a tough situation or, like Alex, move forward into the rest of your exciting career and life, you need to put first things first. At the start, you have to get clear in your mind that the time has finally come for you to take care of yourself. You should decide that putting self-care and the twelve actions at the forefront of your daily life are a necessary and deliberate way to give your life positive momentum. If you feel dread or anxiety over the thought of making a change and giving some time and attention to yourself, maybe you're not ready. Don't worry, just keep trying to get yourself mentally prepared.

Good sleep is the second chronological step in your journey toward good health. I'm not talking about one night every week or so, when you go to bed early and sleep soundly through the night, or when you sleep in on the weekends. When I say good sleep, I mean at least seven to eight hours of restorative, healing, satisfying rest, supported and made possible by a solid routine. I strongly believe that you can have the best of everything—but you have to work for it. Preparing for and falling into a solid sleep routine is no exception.

Steps three and four are a healthy diet and a regular practice of exercise—but we'll discuss them in greater detail in other actions in this book.

You may be wondering, *Why didn't you talk about mental clarity or sleep in the first action, MaryRuth?* I held off because I don't think that either of these phases have to be the primary entry point into my program. Everyone has a different approach to their health, so one person might want to try Liquids till Lunch first, while another may feel more comfortable eating healthy foods or attempting to get fifteen minutes of sunshine a day. I don't want to tell you that you absolutely must do one action before another because a particular action might not speak to you, and if it doesn't, you might be tempted to give up on the whole program. You're worth all the positive benefits that come with working through the micro actions every day.

My point is that you'll never achieve *full* self-mastery if you don't accomplish the four overarching phases: mental clarity, sleep, food, and exercise. Understanding and becoming proficient in all of them—no matter how long it takes—is what permits you to move forward every day. Just completing every action every day isn't enough. You have to be deliberate about embracing and gaining control of the four phases. Only then will you experience true and long-term change that alters the DNA of your life.

Deep down, most of us understand that sleep is the foundation on which a solid, healthy life is built, but we don't appreciate or act on that every day. Too many people think of sleep as something they can slot in after they've finished all their work or only when they're caught up on their favorite Netflix series. That was what happened to Alex.

"I only sleep when there is absolutely nothing left to do in my day. I mean, *nothing*. So, I go to bed around 1 or 2 and wake up at 7 or 8."

Alex told me he'd always taken sleep for granted because he had so much research to do, homework to finish, tests to prepare for, and socializing to do with people who could help him get ahead. He'd been a striver and a workaholic since he was in elementary school, and those qualities had gotten him everywhere in life. However, all those achievements came at the expense of laying a foundation that would allow him to feel his best and truly thrive for decades in his career and life.

Alex was in his thirties now, and, as far as your brain is concerned, that's not young. Research shows that, starting around age twenty-seven, cognitive decline begins. Abstract reasoning, problem solving, and brain speed take a big hit right at the time that people like Alex are working harder than they have in their entire lives, staying up later at their jobs, or partying till dawn. Too many young adults think that sleep is something to catch up on during the weekends, or that a habitual lack of sleep won't affect them in the long term. Unfortunately, it will.

Health Benefits of Sleep

I read an anonymous quote recently that stated, "There are two types of tired; one is a dire need for sleep, and the other is a dire need for peace." There's a great deal of truth in these words, and anyone who's suffered intense physical or emotional trauma and lost sleep because of it—like I did when I lost my dad and brother—knows the profound exhaustion that comes with pain. I'm not saying that lack of peace is exclusive to an emotionally painful situation, though. Throughout my three full-term pregnancies, and especially the last one with my twins, my body never really felt at peace. I was thrilled to be pregnant, but I woke up two or three times a night to go to the bathroom and

MOVE FORWARD EVERY DAY

Many people like to unwind before bed with a glass of wine or a few beers but, while alcohol might help you fall asleep, it also disrupts your REM sleep and causes you to wake up far less refreshed. The effects are most pronounced in the second half of the night, when you're into the most healing part of sleep. The more you drink, the worse the effects are, so if you do drink, try to keep it at a minimum, and don't do it every night.

had to put an alarm clock across my room so I wouldn't sleep through it. I physically suffered through my emotional happiness, and that imbalance erupted in night after night of chaotic sleep.

What I'm saying is that there's really no boundary between mind and bodily exhaustion. Sleep *is* peace. It mediates the external stressors in life and gives your body an inner harmony that allows it to handle life's endless pressures.

Specifically, when you sleep, your blood pressure goes down, giving your cardiovascular system a time to rest. Your heart beats softly, your breathing slows, and what was once a raging river during the day quiets down to a gently flowing stream. When you don't sleep enough, your blood pressure stays high and, over time, that puts you at a greater risk for heart disease and stroke.

Sleep influences your hormones as well, and when you fall into REM sleep—the deepest, most restorative stage of your night's rest—your endocrine system activates. The endocrine system is the collection of glands that make hormones for metabolism, growth, reproduction, and more. At night, these glands release growth hormone, luteinizing hormone, and prolactin, all of which grow, repair, and develop cells and tissues. Lack of sleep increases the level of the stress hormone cortisol, which in turn causes your cells to resist the effects of insulin. Insulin instructs your fat, muscle, and liver cells how to absorb glucose (or blood sugar), so if that cell–insulin connection is blocked, blood-sugar levels will remain elevated. What disease does consistently high blood-sugar levels indicate you have? Type 2 diabetes. In fact, research shows that adults who sleep an average of six hours a night are 1.7 times more likely to have diabetes compared to people who sleep seven or eight hours a night. Even worse, adults who average five or fewer hours of sleep a night are 2.5 times more likely to have diabetes.

As if hormonal havoc wasn't enough to disrupt any peace you might find in your life, a chronic or persistent lack of sleep also lowers your immunity. A strong, responsive immune system is vital for preventing and battling illnesses as minor as the common cold and as major at COVID-19. When you sleep, levels of the stress hormones adrenaline and noradrenaline and a molecule called *prostaglandin* decrease. These substances prevent your immune system's T cells—which are central to the fight against germs—from functioning at their highest level. The natural suppression of your body's stress hormones during sleep also causes you to feel less anxious during the day. If you don't get enough sleep, stress hormone levels remain high, which increases the likelihood you'll exhibit a fight-or-flight response in reaction to perceived or real threats. I'm sure you've experienced this phenomenon. Think of those really awful early mornings after you've been up half the night with a crying baby or insomnia. You crawl out of bed to get ready for work and you stumble into the kitchen to pour yourself a cup of coffee. Your husband is standing there. He looks at you and says, "What happened to you? You don't look so good!"

ROAR!! You bite his head off.

It's okay; you're not being rude. You're defensive and reactive because lack of sleep kept your stress hormones up.

When you get enough deep, restorative sleep, though, not only do you calm down, but your brain function levels out. Your mind sharpens, and your memory, focus, and response times improve. You stop making mistakes and your judgment becomes better. Maybe you don't send that angry email to your coworker and realize you can talk to him face-to-face the next day, or maybe you don't make a rash decision to buy a new iPhone you don't really need. Maybe, like Alex did after a week of good sleep, you check an important research project one last time and see an error that changes the entire outcome for the better.

The negative effects of a lack of sleep are cumulative: in terms of brain function and emotional and physical well-being, three nights of less than seven hours is equivalent to one night of no sleep. We all know how terrible a sleepless night feels and how

MOVE FORWARD EVERY DAY

Magnesium is one of the often-overlooked supplements that can make a huge difference in how you sleep at night. Anxious people or individuals who regularly experience insomnia or restless, interrupted sleep often have a magnesium deficiency. Yet most blood work won't reveal your magnesium levels. Magnesium works by increasing your body's levels of the neurotransmitter GABA, which promotes relaxation and good sleep. Magnesium also helps regulate your body's stress response and, with a more balanced approach to stress, you'll definitely sleep better. The recommended dosage is anywhere from 100–350 mg taken right before bed. Some people start with the lowest possible dose and see how it affects their sleep, but, as always, you should check with your doctor first.

long it takes you to recover physically and mentally, so think about that when you choose to stay up late or wake up before your body is truly ready. You *need* to get enough sleep on a regular, consistent basis.

The positive benefits of getting enough sleep are cumulative as well. One night of great rest may cause you to feel so good that you ask for that promotion you've been dreaming of. Or one week of feeling refreshed and relaxed may cause you to start exercising again or make a habit of calling your friends more often. Or, if you're Alex, one month of making sleep a priority rather than an afterthought will cause your advisor to text me and say, *He's a changed man. I've never seen anyone so level-headed and professional with truly great self-composure.*

What *Is* Good Sleep?

Most doctors and scientists will tell you that you need a minimum of seven to eight hours of sleep to be able to function at your optimal level the next day and for your body to be able to grow, repair, and heal properly overnight. This was true for almost every client I ever had, and it's definitely true for me. I need about eight hours of sleep every single night to be able to feel energized, positive, and balanced, and to run my company, raise my children, work out, cook dinner, and be a good friend and a loving wife and daughter. Without eight hours of sleep, I also can't do the hard work of looking at the world and my community and seeing how I can make a real contribution, treat my fellow citizens the way I'd like to be treated, and work toward a better tomorrow. These are hugely important tasks in the tough times we live in, but I'm committed to them as much as my personal priorities, and I can't do any of them well without good sleep.

I've had clients and friends who can sleep between six and seven hours a night, though, and still perform to their highest-functioning capacity. I think of someone I know named Alysha, who works at a nonprofit that advocates for housing equality. She feels so passionate about what she does that she wakes up in the morning fired up and ready to go. Even though her three young children run her ragged when she's not at work, she's found her calling and is putting so much good out in the world, she feels alive. Less than seven hours of sleep just works for her because she's always in her zone. She's positive, treats her body well—working out five times a week and drinking plenty of water—and eats healthy food. I wouldn't dream of telling her to sleep more because the formula she's found works beautifully for her life.

If you've settled into your zone like Alysha, just be careful not to take the idea of sleeping less too far. I know there are some of you out there who swear up and down that you're just fine with six hours of sleep or less, but that really only works for the short term. In the long term, you need more sleep than that, and research backs this up. A sleep deprivation study published in 2003 in *Sleep* looked at forty-eight adults who were permitted to sleep a maximum of only six hours a night for two weeks. By the tenth day, their cognitive performance was as poor as people who were kept up for two nights in a row without *any* sleep. But here's what's so interesting: these same semifunctioning people thought they were doing just fine! They had absolutely no idea they were so impaired.

A good night's sleep should be one where you wake feeling refreshed, and you're not sleepy during the day. If you've slept well, you have mental clarity and, for the sixteen to seventeen hours that remain in the circle that represents your day, you're happy with the amount of energy you have. Your energy might wane a little sometimes during the day, but you know how to rally. You're in your zone, and the internal fire burning inside you matches the external energetic forces that act on you throughout the day.

If you regularly depend on more than one cup of coffee in the morning to wake up, that's not a good sign. For many of you, coffee is energizing and satisfying, and you can't imagine your morning without that warm cup of therapy. There is nothing wrong with that, and a regular dose of pure comfort is *great*. The Food and Drug Administration (FDA) also says that anything under 400 mg of caffeine (roughly four cups of coffee) is not detrimental to your health, but I always told my clients that if you need more than one cup to come out of what feels like a stupor, that's a red flag that you're not sleeping enough. Your body always sends clear signs when something is off, so don't ignore your body and the signals it shares with you. Depending on a stimulant to operate on a basic level during the day is, without a doubt, a sign that you're not getting enough sleep.

Don't Forget Your Pregame

If you're getting the right amount of satisfying sleep at night, you need to have what I call a pregame. A pregame is a strict series of steps that allow you to prepare for bed and go to sleep at the right time for you. You have to be diligent about your pregame, but to really enjoy it, I recommend making it fun.

You can create any structured routine you want, but here's what I do. Just like I did for Alex, I have a circle that's divided up into all the hours within a twenty-four-hour period. I like to get up at 6 a.m. and need at least eight hours of sleep, so I've marked 10 p.m. as my bedtime. From that, I work backwards.

I know it takes me fifteen minutes to get ready for bed, so I've indicated 9:30 on the circle as the time I absolutely must walk into my bathroom and put on my pajamas. When I was single, this was much easier; there were fewer tasks to do and no toys to pick up. Now, I have those things plus my husband, who I want to watch TV with and talk to at night. But I know sleep is my foundation, so, no matter what's still not picked up or what we've queued up on Netflix, I walk up the stairs precisely at 9:30 p.m. unless we're out that night.

Here's where I've elevated my nighttime routine into a ritual. I shut my bathroom door, dim the lights to a soothing level, and slip on a pair of soft, comfortable PJs. I wash my face carefully and deliberately and rub an essential oil—usually lavender, which helps me sleep—onto the bottom of my feet. I check to make sure my alarm is set and slide into bed no later than 9:45. My husband comes upstairs, and we talk and catch up for a little bit. We're always laughing about something that happened that day. No later than 10 p.m., I turn off the light. My body and mind have fallen seamlessly into that healing, ritualized repetition, and, most of the time, I'm asleep within two minutes.

When I first drew my circle, I also marked 7 p.m. with a line. That was three hours before I wanted my head to hit my pillow, so that's when I would plan to finish my dinner. It takes your organs three to four hours to digest food, and if there's food in your belly when you fall asleep, your body has to shift its energy toward digestion rather than toward cellular growth, repair, and regeneration. If there's absolutely no way you can stop eating three to four hours before bed, don't go to sleep hungry. Instead, have a light, more easily digestible meal that's balanced between water-dense and nutrient-dense foods.

I know many of you push your bedtime later and later because you want to watch TV, catch up on emails, or have a little fun after a long, hard day, but you can't sabotage yourself by cutting back on sleep. There is so much power in putting your bedtime on autopilot; I promise that within a week of being deliberate and diligent about winding down and getting to bed, you'll start to see the micro action of sufficient rest connect with the macro action of moving forward in your life. Nothing feels better than a good night's sleep, and the more you do it, the more momentum and energy you'll have to do the things you love. You'll also see that when you get up earlier, you somehow seem to get so much more done than when you try to do those same things late at night.

I find that people are *very* strict about other actions in my program, yet they tend to gloss over the issue of sleep. They'll direct-message me to proudly say, *I'm doing Liquids till Lunch for thirty days. I've cleaned out all the cereal from my pantry and bought a juicer. When the thirty days are up, I'm rewarding myself!* But I have never, ever gotten a similar direct message about sleep. It's

MOVE FORWARD EVERY DAY

You should always aim to fall asleep or be in a state of deep relaxation by 10 p.m., and not just because waking up early, before most of the rest of the world comes alive, grants you the fabulous feeling of having a head start on your day. The hours after 10 are also prime time for your hormones.

Right around 10 p.m., your metabolism starts to shift in response to the melatonin that your pineal gland has produced in preparation for sleep. If you're not asleep or in a state of deep relaxation, this metabolic shift won't happen. And if it doesn't, your body can't fully enter its cellular repair-and-restore mode.

Melatonin also influences the release of human growth hormone, which helps your body burn fat, repair collagen, regenerate tissue, improve bone density, and boost immunity. There are three distinct spikes in growth hormone (hGH)—one at 10 p.m., another at 2 a.m., and the last at 4 a.m. If you're awake during those hours, the growth hormone won't be as effective performing these functions, so, again, you'll deprive your body of the vital repair and growth it needs.

time to change that. Sleep is everything, and while sometimes it may be hard to prioritize or ease into it, I promise you can with a whole lot of perseverance.

Perseverance

Not only is there a ton of research out there about the negative health effects of sleep loss, there also isn't a single grown-up in the world who'd doesn't love an amazing night of rest. Yet according to a survey the Centers for Disease Control (CDC) conducted in 2016, more than one-third of Americans say they regularly don't get enough sleep. I've talked a lot about how too many people don't prioritize sleep, but I don't think that's the full story. I also think that putting sleep first and foremost in your life and structuring your day around it requires consistent work. And work is, well, really, really hard for a lot of people.

Moving forward in life is a process, though, and you can't just close your eyes and hope that optimism and inspiration will make your dreams come true. You can't be passive about the things your body, mind, and soul need most, which means you simply can't be relaxed about your need for sleep. You absolutely, positively must work and work to make it a regular part of your life.

One of my favorite quotes is "Perseverance is the hard work you do after you get tired of doing the hard work you already did." Creating a regular practice of getting good sleep involves nothing but perseverance. I know it's easy to fall into a stupor scrolling through your social media instead of getting up to put

MOVE FORWARD EVERY DAY

The foods you eat—especially in the hours before you go to bed—may help or harm your sleep quality depending on how acidic or alkaline they are. White bread and pasta, sugars, animal proteins (including fish), sugary foods and drinks, dairy, and margarine are acidic, and they lower the pH level of your body. The way your body filters out acid and stabilizes its pH level is through perspiration and urination, and you are most acidic at around 2 a.m. So, if you regularly wake up in the middle of the night to go to the bathroom, that may be a sign that you're eating too many acidic foods.

You can combat acid buildup by replacing acidic foods with alkaline foods. These include dark, leafy greens, certain fruits, beans, millet, quinoa, nuts, seeds, avocado, olive oil, and many more foods. These will help halt an acid buildup during the day, and that will help you sleep like a baby at night.

on your pajamas, and I understand it feels so much easier to lie in bed with the TV on than turn it off and face the anxiety that sometimes keeps you up at night. The point is that, even when you're tired of it, hard work involves doing the same thing over and over again till you break through and it becomes second nature. Perseverance is the strength of character that comes from all that hard work. It's a quality to be proud of; you were strong, and you had drive. You did it, and now you can sleep.

I hear from customers all the time who complain that they've always been terrible sleepers. They sometimes even dread going to bed because that means they'll toss and turn till 1 a.m. or, worse, be up all night. *What's the point of even trying?* they'll direct-message me. *I'd rather just stay up with my husband and have a glass of wine.* Don't do it. If you're like this, you're already in a situation that's not ideal, so don't make it worse by going to bed late. Try magnesium, and if that doesn't work, try hemp oil from hemp seeds, which helps reduce anxiety and prolong periods of sleep. Exercise during the day so your body starts to wind down at night. Dim the lights and turn off all the screens around you. Go see the doctor and dig deeply for a root cause. A friend of mine slept fitfully for years, averaging about five hours a night. After five years of searching for the cause, he discovered he had an autoimmune disease. He treated it and eliminated his insomnia, and now he looks forward to getting in bed at night. Do anything and everything to get your rest, and never, ever stop trying. Persevere through the hard times and force yourself to go to bed by 10 p.m. so you can maybe—just maybe—fall asleep and be well rested the next day. Work *harder* to make sleep a priority. Once you do, a lot of answers about life's different challenges will unfold for you.

8.

Fifteen Minutes of Stretching

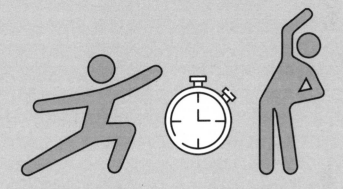

Many of my clients came to me after a lifetime of being out of shape. They had spent their childhoods dreading gym class because they felt humiliated in front of their classmates, or they refused to go to the community pool with their friends because they would be seen in a bathing suit. These experiences might seem minor, but they scarred a lot of people, especially women like Michelle.

Michelle had come from a stable, happy family, and she was especially close to her big sister. But while she'd always carried a little bit of extra weight, her sister was very thin. Her sister was a cheerleader, and Michelle avoided football games. Her sister ran track. Michelle couldn't run a mile. Her sister had competed at the state level in gymnastics. Michelle couldn't do a cartwheel.

Even though Michelle's family loved her and supported all her interests and activities—particularly writing, which she excelled at—her self-esteem was always low. She just wasn't like her popular, athletic sister, and she constantly felt inadequate because of it. After college, she dated, then later married a man who sometimes joked about her weight. She had jobs with bosses who belittled her in meetings, and, when we first met, she consistently downplayed her accomplishments.

"Something I wrote got published online," she told me, "but I know it isn't very good."

I worked with Michelle for a full year, texting her daily to help keep her on a healthy diet and encourage her to do the twelve actions every day to the best of her ability. Slowly, my program started to click with her, and midway through the year, Michelle lost ten pounds and registered for a charity walk. A month after the walk, she quit the job she hated. By the end of the year, she'd asked her husband to move out, and he did. She bought a new bathing suit, and she and her sister went on a cruise.

Of all the incredible accomplishments Michelle made in the time I knew her, though, there was one that stuck in my mind the most. It sounded so simple, but to Michelle, it was profound. Just this one little act of self-mastery chipped away at a lifetime of low self-esteem and signaled to her that her life had opened up, expanded, and blossomed in ways that impacted her body, mind, and spirit.

"I touched my toes for the first time in my life," she said. "I thought I'd never be able to do that."

Bit by bit and inch by inch, Michelle had moved forward that year. When her fingers reached her toes, they might have just made the lightest touch. To Michelle, that one small accomplishment signaled a giant leap.

Become the Cause, Not the Effect

Michelle had spent over three decades being reactive and feeling one step behind everyone and everything in her life. When her then-boyfriend had asked her to marry him, she'd known it was a mistake, but she'd figured, *No one else will ever want me.* When her boss asked her to sign on for a six-month project she hated the sound of, she accepted it, thinking, *I'm too tired to interview for a new job.* Yet one simple action helped her self-confidence skyrocket. Sure, it took a concerted effort for her to get there and, just like her charity walk, she'd had to put in the time and effort every single day. But trying to touch her toes wasn't grueling work that required expensive equipment or even made her break a sweat. She could stretch anywhere, almost anytime, and she did it fifteen minutes a day, following my recommendation.

"I stretched when I was on conference calls at work," she said. "I'd put on my headset, stand up, and stretch any way that felt natural. No one in the cubes near me even noticed."

I work stretching into my life in a similar way to Michelle. When one of my older boys wakes up in the morning, I walk into his room, but I don't get him out of his crib right away. I hand him a toy or a book, give him a big kiss on the head, and talk to him about the day ahead. Then I begin to stretch. I roll my neck around and let it hang low. I sweep my arms over my head, drop my shoulders, and lean to the left, then right. I sit on the ground and extend my legs out into a "V" position, then turn slightly and lean down over each leg. I hold these stretches for as long as I like, breathing and talking steadily the whole time.

I do something similar in the kitchen, too. If I'm waiting for water to boil on the stove or something in the oven to finish cooking, I don't always check my phone or look around the kitchen for dishes to put away. Instead, I try to relax and, for as long as I can, I bend and stretch.

Stretching in those found minutes gives me a feeling of self-mastery. *I'm* controlling my time rather than what's cooking on the stove controlling it for me. *I'm* managing my son's expectations for the morning instead of him controlling how the day is going to proceed. He still comes out of his bed happy and well-loved, and I leave his room with a body and mind that feel better because I've taken care of them. When Michelle started stretching, she stopped feeling like she was a hostage to her overweight, anxious body, nor did she feel trapped by a boring conference call. That half hour call was *her* time to improve her body.

Stretching is a real litmus test for where you are in your life. How and when you fit it into your day can help you answer the questions: Do you control your time, or do others? Are you organized and on top or are you reactive to chaos, letting people and events overwhelm you? For fifteen minutes in a twenty-four-hour period, stretching allows you to be the cause rather the effect. For that tiny increment of time every day, you can manage the mental and physical blocks that can prevent you from moving forward by taking real *action*.

We all complain about not having enough personal time, but I think self-care is especially hard for caregivers or people whose jobs involve an intense, direct responsibility for the well-being of another person or persons. Nurses, doctors, teachers, parents, and many others spend every waking hour laboring through an endless series of often life-or-death tasks that require immediate attention. In a quiet moment between all those overwhelming responsibilities, it's helpful to realize that you can stop, stretch,

MOVE FORWARD EVERY DAY

There are many different categories of stretching, including passive, ballistic, static, and dynamic. If you haven't trained at a high level in a sport or seen a physical therapist or trainer, you may be unfamiliar with these terms, so let me define them for you.

- STATIC STRETCHING: This is the most common and basic form of stretching, in which you remain in a muscle-lengthening pose (like touching your toes) for anywhere between ten and thirty seconds. It's used to improve general flexibility.

- ACTIVE STRETCHING: In this technique, you hold a stretch while simultaneously contracting the muscle against that same stretch. For example, you might bend your leg at the knee and extend your foot back toward your glute. Instead of holding your foot, as you would in a passive stretch, stay balanced on one foot with your other leg tight, feeling the lengthening and strengthening in the front of your thigh.

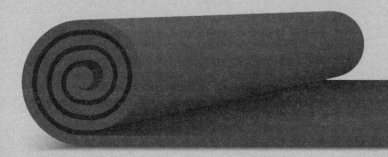

- BALLISTIC STRETCHING: **This is a static stretch with an added and repeated bounce to force a muscle beyond its normal range of motion. For example, if you lean over with your hands toward your toes, then bob gently up and down, you're implementing a ballistic stretch.**

- PASSIVE STRETCHING: **A stretch in which you relax a muscle and then an external force—like a body weight, a strap, gravity, or another person—lengthens the muscle in a fixed, held position. For example, if you're lying on your back with your leg raised, and your trainer pushes it toward you, you're engaging in a passive stretch.**

- DYNAMIC STRETCHING: **This is a slow-moving, con- trolled stretch—repeated ten to twelve times—that often requires a degree of balance. Used by athletes and trainers to improve range of motion, it's not held, like a static stretch is. One example is the "zombie walk," where you hold your arms out at a 90-degree angle, then extend one leg up toward your fingers, then another. Walk forward slowly the whole time, just like a zombie!**

and transform yourself into an agent of personal change. I promise you'll experience a tangible mental shift that tells you that you are in charge. You have power.

You aren't tricking your mind or altering your reality when you begin to think this way. You're simply shifting your framework into a more positive place that's all-around better for you and the people around you. The late author Robert Collier wrote, "Success is the sum of small efforts, repeated day in and day out." This is the concept of healing through repetition, of course. Turning time that would normally be allocated 100 percent to someone or something else into time for you is a small effort that yields immediate success—and often a much better mood. And the best thing is that you can do it day after day *for free*. Don't worry, you'll still be there for your friends, family, and commitments. I'm giving *more* to my children when I stand in their rooms and stretch. When I stretch while I'm talking to my friend on the phone, I'm not distracted from her or her needs. Instead, that captured moment, when I've deliberately stopped to listen, gives her more of me. Simultaneously, I am also giving back more to myself.

Health Benefits of Stretching

When it comes to flexibility and range of motion, no two people are alike. There are some people who will absolutely never be able to do a backbend, and there are others who could hold themselves up in the wheel position for a few minutes, no problem. People who are more limber tend to have more collagen and elastin—the protein fibers that help give skin its structure—within their joints and ligaments. While a relatively inflexible person won't magically become hyperflexible after stretching regularly for a month, the many health benefits of stretching prove that it's one of the fundamental parts of a good exercise routine.

The principle behind stretching is that it pushes your muscles, tendons, and ligaments from a state of inactivity to one of growth and production. The process may not be comfortable—a good stretch can feel like your muscles are on fire—but it is growth through pain. As you force your body into a difficult space, stretching beyond its limits, your stem cells begin to produce more protein, including collagen and elastic. Over time, the stretch will begin to feel less painful as you add length to your muscle fibers.

Anyone who's ever woken up in the morning and stretched their arms into the air (so, pretty much, all of us) knows that stretching helps wake you up. After a night of relative inactivity, your muscles are often stiff, and stretching helps you work out the kinks. But that's not the whole story. When you're lying down, especially over a few hours, the fluid in your body—including lymph and blood—pools in your lower back. Stretching massages that fluid back into circulation.

Stretching helps increase blood flow to the muscles at any time of day as well. If you feel sleepy at 4 p.m., try stretching instead of getting a cup of coffee or tea. You might be surprised at how much more awake and alive you feel. Not only do you increase the circulation of blood to your muscles, you also improve the distribution of nutrients throughout your tissues. By stretching, you are literally nourishing your body on a cellular level.

Stretching also helps improve your posture. I remember the first time I met Michelle. I immediately noticed there was a noticeable rounding to the middle of her back, and her shoulders rose up at an unnatural angle toward her ears. She hunched when she was sitting or standing, and her poor posture gave her a look of overall defeat. What was really happening is that the muscles in her back were tense, forcing her body to bend to overcompensate. I don't want to blame Michelle's low self-esteem or aversion to exercise for this slouch; she also spent most of her day sitting in

MOVE FORWARD EVERY DAY

Contrary to what many of us learned in gym class, you shouldn't do static stretches before a hard workout. A comprehensive review of 104 studies on exercise and stretching concluded that static stretching before an exercise lessens the strength, power, and explosive performance you might attain. Instead, try to warm up for ten to fifteen minutes before exercise with dynamic stretches or a light activity like jumping jacks, lunges, or jogging in place. Then, after you finish your workout, you can stretch any way that feels good to your tired muscles.

a chair staring at a computer, so her body settled into a particular position that required less effort. Stretching can counteract this. When you stretch any part of your body—but especially your torso, hips, and arms—you relax your tight muscles, helping your body fall back into its natural alignment.

Stretching may have preventative benefits as well. Research shows that when you stretch you are better able to maintain balance. A 2012 study looked at forty-two people who were asked to stand on a small, moveable platform called a *stabilometer*. The subjects who stretched for thirty minutes before the test were able to balance longer than those who didn't. Scientists believe that's because stretching allowed their muscles to learn how to coordinate and work out their response to the platform's instability, and they made small adjustments to help them stay upright. Along the same lines, stretching may also help prevent injuries by putting you in the right mindset before a physical activity. When you limber up your body even a little bit, you start to focus on the muscles you'll be exercising and the range of motion you'll have to move through. This is pure bodily awareness and muscle memory; you're in touch with your body, and you have an innate road map for the work it does.

Finally, stretching has been proven to help lower stress levels. When we're exposed to a real threat or when we're consumed with worry that something bad might happen (even if, chances are, it won't), adrenaline surges through our veins, and our bodies get ready to deploy their fight-or-flight response. Our muscles tense up as thoughts race through our brains. After even a short period of time, this can really cause your body to hurt. Stretching can help! As your muscles extend, the tension dissipates and blood flow increases. Within your body, you create an openness and receptivity, freeing good energy that has profound implications on both the emotional and physical levels.

Openness and Stagnation

Many of you who practice yoga understand the concept of openness. In hundreds of asanas, or yoga poses, the goal is to allow the body to unfold and become receptive to the energetic forces in the world. As a muscle or a body part broadens, stretches, and opens, your interior energy ceases to stagnate. It dislodges, then flows freely within you and radiates outside you, allowing you to achieve a peaceful balance between the dynamics of the outside world and those inside your body. In upward facing dog, for example, you extend your legs behind you and place your hands under you, then rise up, letting your shoulders drop, your chin rise, your chest expand, and your heart open. Your ribs seem to part, creating a sense of freedom across your upper body. In butterfly pose, you sit upright, placing the inner soles of your feet together and letting your knees fall to the side as if you're opening a book. As your inner thighs and groin stretch, you find a spaciousness in your hips.

You don't have to practice yoga to appreciate these sensations. Many of us experience the quiet emotional release of our muscles lengthening and our fluids flowing when we stretch, yet we've never stopped to describe it. Yoga does, however, and for many people, the description is eye opening. It's a relief to know they can put a name to the powerful physical feelings and emotions of the letting go that comes with stretching.

Emotional blocks are often described in physical terms. When you're overburdened, you have the weight of the world on your shoulders. If you're worried about something, you have a knot in your stomach. If you can't find the right words to describe something, you have a lump in your throat. These scenarios that cross the mind/body barrier aren't limited to negative or traumatic experiences. When you're excited about something, you may have courage coursing through your veins.

One of the central concepts of traditional Chinese medicine (TCM) is something called *Qi* (pronounced *chee*). Qi is the vital energy that affects everything about who we are, and it encompasses the external forces around us as well as the internal energetic forces like illness, body chemistry, and thoughts and feelings. Qi is believed to stagnate when we're anxious or stressed, and it manifests itself in physical ailments such as depression, mood swings, digestive upset, or painful periods.

People who work in TCM or in bodywork practices like acupuncture or massage have identified and mapped out these places within the body where Qi stagnates and emotional barriers are stored. For example, "fear of doing" is lodged in the center of the back, while "shame" is believed to be stored just to the side of the armpits. When a practitioner works on your body, they may target these problem areas, trying to loosen the knots that are the physical manifestations of your pain or stress. A massage therapist will rub your sore shoulders or back, creating heat in the muscles, increasing blood flow through them, relaxing them, and reducing nerve compression within them. An acupuncturist inserts a tiny needle into the skin, which stimulates nerves, causing them to send a signal to your brain. In response, your brain releases endorphins—neurochemicals that act like painkillers—masking pain and giving you a sense of well-being. As endorphins flood the area that's been bothering you, negative energy dissipates, stagnation decreases, and healing begins.

These concepts come up in traditional medicine as well. In *The Body Keeps the Score*, Bessel van der Kolk describes how the body doesn't forget emotional or physical trauma and stores that pain within us—sometimes for a lifetime. People who've experienced sexual abuse, for example, often have great difficulty opening their hip muscles and joints and may experience pain in them. When they stretch or try hip-opening poses in yoga—such as happy baby or butterfly—they often resist them, then they break out in tears when they finally try it and feel the pressure release in those tightly wound muscles.

Michelle hadn't been sexually abused, but her negative body image made her slouch and subsequently experience back pain. In contrast, her confident older sister had an almost perfect posture, with dropped shoulders, a natural arch, and almost no tension in her back.

Van der Kolk writes that traumatized people can alleviate these emotional and physical blocks through bodywork practices. They can dance, do yoga, try acupuncture or massage, or they can gradually, then repeatedly, assume whatever position makes them uncomfortable and stretch those muscles. That's right; counteracting energetic stagnation and working against pain and trauma can be as simple as stretching for fifteen minutes a day.

Stretching may hurt at first, but that initial pain recedes when you work at it, allowing healing and resilience to set in. You get your fluids moving. You nourish your tissues. Just like acupuncture, stretching sends a signal to the brain to release endorphins, so you mask pain and boost pleasure. You start to wake up. You activate your cells, allowing them to produce proteins. Your wounds heal as your emotional blocks loosen, and your heart and body open up.

Stagnation isn't just an emotional response. Those who haven't exercised in weeks, months, or even years, sometimes hit physical barriers when they try to start an exercise routine. Their muscles scream in pain, their hearts race, or their joints ache so much that they simply have to stop.

"I didn't exercise from the time I was eighteen—when I went to my last high school gym class—through most of my awful marriage in my twenties," Michelle told me. "I only started right around when I turned thirty and decided to get divorced. And when I first got going, I couldn't do *anything*."

Michelle had joined a gym and tried her first Zumba class. She got so winded that she left the class midway through and stepped on the treadmill. When she developed a cramp in her side, she started to cry and rushed back to the changing room, vowing she'd never go back to the gym. Luckily, good friends convinced her to try a free intro session with a trainer.

"That changed everything for me," she said, "because during that session, all we did was stretch."

If you're overweight, have a health challenge, have been in an accident, or—like Michelle—are going through a divorce and have life challenges—stretching can provide the bare minimum for your body but still deliver profound effects. Stretching can give you a sense of freedom if you're experiencing positive pressure from your career goals. If you've given yourself a pass on exercise for weeks or months because you're just not in the mood (and that's totally okay), stretching can get you back into your groove. Two sessions of stretching with her trainer were enough for Michelle's body to awaken from the stagnation she'd felt for years, and, soon, he convinced her to sign up for the charity walk. While she was training for it, she started eating a healthy diet and worked out with weights a few times a week.

For Michelle, stretching was a critical beginning; it opened doors and showed her body and mind that bigger, better things lay ahead. It was the cure for decline and stagnation, and even though it seemed so simple, it was the perfect micro action that added up bit by bit and moved her life forward.

Grief Is Expanding

When I was in my sophomore year of college, something happened in my life that I haven't talked about very much. About seven years after my dad died suddenly and six months before my brother passed away, a good friend whom I'd met in college and had worked with in the intramural referee department there was murdered. He was only nineteen years old, and he was on the dean's list, studying to become an accountant. He was tall, handsome, charismatic, and loved by *everyone*.

My friend had ended up at a small party in Brooklyn after a night out with a few friends. He didn't have enough money to get a car back to the place where he was staying in New Jersey, so he stayed out longer than he normally would. It's still unclear what happened over the course of the night, but at around 4 a.m., the neighbors in the quiet, residential neighborhood where the party had been heard shots. Not long after, he was found dead, face down on a yellow blanket in someone's driveway. Five bullets were in his body, and he'd been severely beaten.

The case made national headlines immediately; the suspects were young and well off, the possible motives were bizarre, and the evidence was spotty. A lot of my friends were interviewed by the police during the long investigation. As the weeks and months passed, the press called again and again for interviews and, in almost every conversation I had at school, my friend's name came up. Day in and day out, grief and trauma suffocated us all. The police didn't arrest anyone for his murder for over a year, so we felt no sense of closure or justice.

Six months after my friend's murder, my younger brother, Daniel, passed away suddenly.

That one-two punch of trauma hung over me for years after that, lodging in my body and making my heart muscles ache.

MOVE FORWARD EVERY DAY

Everyone grieves in a different way—and there is absolutely no wrong approach—but one of the methods that many experts recommend and that I've found helpful is to set aside a time each day dedicated to grieving. It can be five minutes or twenty, but you should do nothing but *feel* in these moments. Cry, mourn, punch your pillow, look at photographs, or—quite the opposite—reflect on all the good things that grief has brought you. No emotion is bad. Think of this as emotional stretching; you're putting yourself into a hard, uncomfortable place in order to grow stronger—and you will.

If you spent most of your life angry at your mother who's just passed, that anger is completely fine, and you should not be ashamed of it. When your dedicated time is up, move on to your next task, doing your best to focus your attention on the present. The goal is to think of grief as an action. Grief wants to move out of your body, and that's why talking about it helps immensely. It's a dynamic process you act on to stretch yourself, work through your pain, and grow into your new life, rather than letting your emotions control you.

When my mom was diagnosed just over a year later with two brain tumors, pain pummeled its way into my life even deeper.

I don't think grief ever fully leaves you. I miss my friend, my dad, and my brother every single day. But I believe grief is about expanding, not shrinking. It's about having more in your life, not less.

My husband, David, and I have always wanted a big family, with children close in age. Ethan and Elliot are just fifteen months apart, and I love that they feel like they might as well be twins. We started trying for another baby not too long after Elliot was born and, on his first birthday, August 19, 2019, I was absolutely thrilled to discover I was pregnant.

Weeks later, I got even better news: I was pregnant with fraternal twins.

David and I were so excited, and I remember catching him looking at me over dinner, then starting to smile and laugh. We booked our doula. We planned how we'd squeeze two cribs into Elliot's room and move Elliot into Ethan's. I put ultrasound photos on my desk at work, and I started to inventory all my old baby stuff. Right about my thirteenth week of pregnancy, when my morning sickness was really hitting me hard, David went away for a ten-day business trip. I didn't think a thing of it because I had so much to look forward to.

A few days into his trip, I woke up at 5 a.m. and realized I was having a miscarriage. (This was my third miscarriage: 2013—twins; 2014—singleton; and 2019—twins.)

I called David, and when he answered, I started crying. When he hung up, I fed and dressed my boys, survived the day, and then went to bed that night. I woke up the next morning and decided to stretch and stick to my usual routine. I'd learned from the deaths of my friend, my dad, and my brother that it's especially powerful and healing during times of loss to keep up a routine if possible. I also knew that the loss doesn't have to shrink your life. It's just the opposite. Grief can expand it. Through the pain, you can grow into the person you're meant to be.

When I first found out I was pregnant with twins that August, I started to work the twelve actions of my program harder and better than I ever had before. I began getting up an hour earlier than usual to inventory my kitchen, take my vitamins, pack lunches, and stretch. After work and on the weekends, I organized my house better than a professional could. Every evening at 5:30, I exercised, and I was asleep by 10 p.m. without fail. The knowledge that my job as a mother was going to double took me to the next level physically and mentally, right to a place I'd always wanted to go but had never been able to reach before. I was so happy with my life, and when I had the miscarriage and the twins were gone, no one could take away the place I'd gotten to. I was in a good position because of them. I was still right there with all I had gained from carrying them for thirteen weeks, and knowing I'd reached the top of my game, I couldn't go back. My grief had expanded me, and the loss of those babies was not in vain. They gave me a huge gift and prepared me for my next twin pregnancy in 2020.

When you take that first, fundamental step toward an exercise routine by adding stretching to your life, imagine that this physical practice will expand you in a way similar to grief. By pushing yourself beyond a comfortable limit, you may feel pain, but that pain allows you to grow. And once you've grown, no one can take that away from you. You've embarked upon a journey of openness and expansiveness that's the exact opposite of stagnation, and it's all upward from there. Yes, your body and mind might suffer, and your accomplishments might seem petty to everyone else, but they're not. When Michelle told me that her proudest accomplishment was touching her toes, I didn't dismiss it. That small stretch had been a huge step for her, and after that she could do almost anything.

Stretching is, in so many ways, symbolic of how great your life can be. You can reach farther. You can dream bigger. You can grasp whatever it is that has felt out of your reach. Don't view your grief of your trauma as a setback even if it feels like it. It's an opening to something bigger that allows you to grow into greatness. Stretch into that new place and enjoy the endorphin release that lets you know you're treating yourself well with self-care. Let your heart open and the tension dissipate from your tired muscles. Stretching has the power to move you forward if you allow it.

9.

Thirty Minutes of Exercise Daily

Walking, jogging, elliptical, or yoga. Whatever will get you moving for thirty minutes.

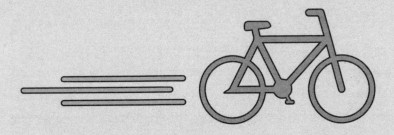

I n any group of friends, there's always one that seems to have it more together than others. The issue isn't necessarily that their house is cleaner or nicer than yours, that they're more beautiful than everyone else, or they've struggled less than you in their lives. They may not be or have any of those things. Instead, they just seem to be doing *something* that gives them genuine confidence and self-mastery. They have a glow to them and a handle on almost every situation, and they're that person that everyone calls first for advice or to share great news.

To all her friends and family, this person was Audrey. Audrey was an attentive listener who always called her friends to check in, and when they reached out and she couldn't talk, she'd text them, *I'll call you back soon.* Even though she had two little children and a demanding job at a restaurant—where she often worked nights—Audrey hosted beautiful dinner parties every few months. She didn't do it to impress anyone; she genuinely liked to cook and entertain because it brought people together. Audrey wasn't perfect. Sometimes she said things that rubbed her friends the wrong way or was late to meetings or appointments, which inconvenienced everyone, including her. But her heart was always in the right place. If a friend was dating a guy who was kind of a jerk, she'd be honest with them and tell them they could do better. And when her children misbehaved, she matter-of-factly, yet lovingly, disciplined them, steering them toward a place that would help them improve.

I ran into Audrey at the grocery store last year, and we started to talk about exercise. While I'd always been athletic and in high school had run cross-country and captained my basketball and lacrosse teams, I told her that exercise had fallen low on my list of priorities since I'd had Ethan and Elliot. I said I was lucky if I could work out three times a week, and while I really wanted to change that, I just hadn't fallen into a good rhythm.

Not Audrey. She worked out at least five times a week for a minimum of thirty minutes a day. She put her workouts into her calendar—and her husband's, too. She scheduled her day around exercise, and while some people thought she bordered on obsessive, I knew she had the right approach. Exercise clearly stood for something crucial in her life. I asked her about it, making it clear I wasn't judging.

"I really admire you for working out so much. How do you do it?"

She looked at me as if she'd been thinking about her answer her whole life. "If I don't exercise," she said, "I'm a much worse friend, daughter, wife, and mom. If I don't exercise, I'm terrible at work. I'm not even that good to *myself*."

There it was in black and white: Audrey was a happier, stronger, calmer, more self-assured and present person because of exercise. Without a shadow of a doubt, working out made each twenty-four-hour period in her life just a little better, and she wasn't going to settle for anything less if she wanted to move forward. Her life and her family were too important.

I believe that for every single person in the world, this philosophy holds true.

Life Is About Choices

Each one of us begins the day with choices to make. Should we choose to get out of bed or push snooze? Should we make a healthy smoothie for breakfast or should we cook up a pile of pancakes? Is today the day to skip work or will we get fired if we do? If you're a single mom with a mortgage, credit card debt, and childcare payments, the decisions you make are probably bigger and more crucial than a high school senior who's on spring break in Florida, but both have responsibilities to themselves and others.

Deep down, most people want to do right by themselves and the world around them. This is essentially the philosophy of natural law: there is an innate moral compass within humans that points us toward positive actions rather than negative ones. This drive toward productive decisions is written into our hearts from the moment we're born and maintains the order of the universe. For example, a plant stretches toward the sun because that energy helps it grow. When it grows and thrives, it can more effectively turn carbon dioxide into oxygen, creating cleaner air for everyone to use. Human beings understand that robbing a bank is wrong. Maybe that instant money delivers a short-term financial gain, but most people don't become thieves because their DNA dictates that doing so would be wrong. They know that stealing traumatizes bank customers and employees, hurts a community, and takes from the hundreds or thousands of people who've entrusted their life savings to that bank.

Exercise corresponds with natural law because our impulse is to move. Sitting on the couch all day cramps your muscles, slows your blood flow, and makes you feel like a slug. Exercise does the opposite. It builds your muscles, clears your brain, wakes you up, and gives you energy, which makes you a better, stronger, healthier, and happier human being who can deliver positive things to your family, friends, and the world. Essentially, exercise puts you into a mental and physical position from which you can help maintain and improve the natural order of the universe.

So, why on earth would you *not* choose to exercise as much as you can?

When Audrey articulated how exercise was a clear-cut choice between positive and negative, a lightbulb went off in my head. *My decision is that simple*, I thought. *I can be a really good mom or a so-so mom. I can run my company like a good leader with my stress under control, or I can fall short of that.* Let me return to an analogy I used earlier in the book. If someone said they'd give you a million dollars if you went to the gym—or nothing if you stayed home—you would jump out of bed in two seconds and sprint to the gym. You'd put on your workout clothes faster than you ever had in your life. Your choice would be crystal clear: instant millionaire or couch potato. That's how Audrey thought of exercise and how I do now, too. I can be a happy person who's optimistic about life or I can feel unmotivated. I can be scared of challenges or I can move forward every day.

We all face different tests—some bigger and more insurmountable than others—so when you're faced with the decision of whether or not to exercise, it's often helpful to utilize short-term thinking. Focusing on a huge goal like losing fifty or one hundred pounds can be scary, especially if the three-mile power walk you took yesterday didn't make your scale budge one pound. Instead, think of what exercise will do for you in *one twenty-four-hour period*. Will it help you be more positive about filing your taxes tonight? Will it give you more energy after a night of bad sleep? Will it prevent you from snapping at your children when they won't do their homework? Successful people usually focus on and master what they're doing with a twenty-four-hour period. They nail it, and that's where the power lies for them.

Long-term goals can feel far away and unreachable, but short-term achievements happen right now. With exercise, you see results fast. Instant energy. Immediate sense of achievement. Knowledge right that second that you've done something good, something natural, and something that will help you put good out into the world. Exercise is that micro step that shifts the direction and advances the momentum of the macro every single day.

Choose the Healthy Path

For maximum health benefits, I recommend you exercise at least thirty minutes a day, five times a week. You should combine muscle-strengthening activities like yoga or lifting weights with aerobic activities like brisk walking, swimming, or gardening, always maintaining a balance between the two kinds of fitness. For example, you could run or take a spin class three days a week and strength train two days. Or do yoga three times a week (with one session more strenuous than the others) and get on the elliptical two days a week.

My advice is in line with what well-respected national and international health organizations recommend. Both the Centers for Disease Control and the American Heart Association say that, every week, you should do a total of 150 minutes of moderate-intensity aerobic activity and two days of muscle-strengthening activities that work all major muscle groups (your legs, arms, hips, abdomen, shoulders, and back). If you choose a really vigorous aerobic exercise like running or spinning, you can cut back your total time to 75 minutes.

This won't come as a surprise to anyone, but the health benefits of regular exercise are huge. Exercise allows your body to shed extra calories, and while many of us grew up believing that more calories burned meant instant weight loss, that's not really the full story. You will have trouble losing weight if you don't exercise *and* eat a healthy diet. The reason for this is that when you diet, your body lowers its basal metabolic rate (BMR) in an effort to metabolize as much energy as possible. It has fewer calories to work with, so it essentially begins a slow, steady burn. When you exercise in addition to eating a healthy diet, you raise your BMR,

MOVE FORWARD EVERY DAY

While everyone should choose the activity that's best suited for them—and, for some people, that's distance running and cycling thirty or so miles—try as hard as possible to stick to shorter-duration athletic activities (around thirty minutes, five times a week). I know some of you might not agree with me, but I worry that if you regularly devote hours a day to exercise, you're probably cutting back on other important things in your life. You may be waking up too early in the morning after sleeping less than seven hours. You may not be taking the time to scan your refrigerator and make grocery lists, or you might be grabbing unhealthy food on the go rather than cooking something healthy that takes a little more time. Doing each of the twelve actions in my program is key to moving forward in your life, and I don't want you to sacrifice one for another. As much as possible, try to maintain a balance among all of them. The power lies in striving to do all twelve actions within a twenty-four-hour period, gradually over time.

turning that low fire into a calorie-scorching inferno. If you keep up a good diet that lowers your blood sugar (that is, one that's not too high in sugar or carbs) and burn more calories that you take in, your body will run more efficiently, and you will lose weight.

Exercise also helps your muscles. When you engage in any kind of physical activity—not just something that's weight bearing—your adrenal system releases hormones that allow your muscles to absorb a greater volume of amino acids. Within twenty-four to forty-eight hours, these absorbed amino acids will begin to grow and repair your muscles—but only if you eat a diet with adequate protein (which should be easy; most Americans consume plenty of protein). Without protein, your muscles can't use amino acids effectively. Once again, just as with weight loss, a healthy diet and exercise work in tandem.

Exercise also improves our bones, especially when we're young. Bones are living tissues, and as you grow up and through your twenties, exercise helps increase their density and mass, making them stronger. But between age thirty and forty, your bones stop growing and they begin to lose their density. If you weren't very physically active in your twenties or early thirties, though, don't worry. It's not too late to stabilize the healthy bones you have. Working out helps maintain bone density and mass, which prevents osteoporosis, a disease in which your bones become more porous and therefore more likely to fracture or break.

Exercise also improves your energy levels. A recent study looked at a group of healthy, disease-free people who complained of feeling fatigued all the time for no apparent reason. The subjects were told to exercise three times a week for a total of six weeks. At the end of that time, they all reported higher levels of energy and less fatigue, regardless of whether they'd chosen to do low-intensity exercises like walking or moderate-intensity work-outs like jogging or swimming. The reason for this across-the-board energy boost may be that, just like stretching, working out causes your body to release endorphins—the "feel good hor-mones" that alleviate pain and promote feelings of well-being. Or it could be that aerobic activity and strength training increase your blood circulation, which moves nutrients into your muscles and nourishes them. Regardless, exercise wakes you up and gets you going, and the study proved that even a moderate amount can help. Never underestimate even ten or twenty minutes of exercise per day if you can't do thirty.

Exercise can improve longevity because it helps prevent and treat chronic diseases like type 2 diabetes and heart disease. Inac-tive people disproportionately experience insulin resistance, a con-dition in which your body doesn't respond to insulin, the hormone that helps regulate your blood sugar. Active people, however, show greater insulin sensitivity. Insulin resistance is an important risk factor for diabetes. There-fore, if you keep up an active lifestyle with a regular exercise routine, you're less likely to develop diabetes.

Exercise lowers your blood pressure and encourages your arteries to dilate more regularly, which improves cardiovascular health and lowers your risk for strokes and heart disease. It also helps increase levels of your HDL, or "good," cholesterol, and flushes your system of LDL, or "bad," artery-clogging cholesterol. High LDL in combination with low HDL is correlated with cardiovascular disease, so people whose cholesterol levels set off a red flag are typically told by their doctors to exercise. Cholesterol levels were one of the first things I looked at when my one-on-one clients got back their blood test results. No one wants to be prescribed cholesterol-lowering drugs, so I always urged clients with poor cholesterol levels to start working out if they didn't do so already and to talk to their doctor.

We've all seen older people who look years, or even decades, younger than they are. While you might think they just got lucky in the genetics department and they might chalk up their youthful looks to good face cream, I can guarantee you that most—if not all—have made exercise a part of their lives. Not only are people who exercise less at risk for many of the chronic diseases that affect their quality of life, they're more likely to shed the excess weight that plagues many people as they age. Their complexion glows because exercise improves circulation to your skin and increases your production of antioxidants, which repair cell damage. Regular exercise has also been shown to improve your sex life. Being happy with your sexual self helps quality of life across the board—from relationships to levels of optimism and positivity. Older people who've made exercise a central part of their routine have gained an advantage, not just physically, but psychologically and mentally. One of the most powerful aspects of exercise is the mental strength it gives you, not just in old age, but for your entire life.

Mental Strength

Audrey's life hadn't always been in great control. In fact, it had spun horribly into chaos when she was sixteen years old and her mom was diagnosed with stage 4 pancreatic cancer. One day, her mom had been a healthy, happy forty-five-year-old. The next day, she was complaining of acid reflux and back pain. Three months later, she was gone, leaving Audrey and her two younger sisters at home with a dad who had depended on his wife for almost everything.

"I don't remember my dad cooking dinner *ever*," Audrey said. "My mom ran all of our lives."

I felt close to Audrey the very first time I met her. My dad had given my family stability and routine. He walked through the door each night, put down his briefcase, took off his coat, and turned on the nightly news so we could watch together. Every summer, he meticulously planned a week's vacation, and whether it was Disney World, Long Beach Island, or Lake Nebo, it was always incredible. When I lost my dad and when Audrey lost her mom, trauma stole that comforting predictability and structure that made life fit like an old glove. Audrey's mom had sewed their Christmas stockings by hand when they were babies. After she passed away, her dad fumbled around the attic for three hours looking for the box where the stockings and ornaments were stored.

Losing your foundation through trauma is an indescribable shock, and your body's usual way of reacting is to freeze up as you brace for the next blow. This can happen even if you receive unexpected *good* news. Think of how a person reacts when they walk into their own surprise birthday party. They usually stop in their tracks, put their hands over their mouth, and don't move until the crowd's finished singing "Happy Birthday." The same happens for some people when they start a new job. They may struggle to figure out what to wear the first day or walk to their desk and stare at it, unsure of where to put their things. The unexpected or new may lead to a total lack of control. Your mind races, struggling to wrap around what to do next. You can't formulate a coherent thought about how to move from one moment to the next. You're unable to move, take action, or do *anything*.

Exercise can combat this mental paralysis. Stuck in a moment where the unforeseen has rendered you unresponsive, you must do the opposite, which is to move. And I don't mean you should slink away, curl up, or run. You need to actively and deliberately engage your body in a way that gives you power. In turn, this physical control grants you mental strength.

Mental strength can mean a lot of things, but think of it as the ability to deal with any kind of pressure or stress. Mental strength is more than having self-awareness or self-mastery. It's the ability to act on those traits, giving you control over your behavior and the way you deal with the world. For Audrey, mental strength was her suggestion to her father that they skip the first Christmas at home without her mom and go on a day trip to the beach—her mom's favorite place in the world—instead. They'd order Chinese food, picnic on a blanket on the sand, then jump in the water to celebrate her mom's life. For me, it was telling my mom that we should go away for a few days after my brother died to a place where we could hike, breathe fresh air, and feel some sense of control over our surroundings before I had to return to college to complete my sophomore year.

If you're that person who's started an exciting new job, yet you find yourself standing at your desk unsure of what to do, don't sit down only to stare at your computer. Start to move around the office, exploring your surroundings and saying hello to your new colleagues. Ask one of them to go out with you for a cup of coffee; just a short walk will help you straighten out your head. Even better, plan to go to the gym at lunch. Exercise does a tremendous amount to provide mental strength and clarity, not just in the short term, but throughout the day.

Exercise improves your sleep quality, a concept that's backed up by scientific research. A two-year study of over 3,000 adults aged eighteen to eighty-five showed that getting 150 minutes of moderate physical activity each week improved the quality of sleep by up to 65 percent. Older participants experienced fewer sleep disruptions like leg cramps, and research subjects of all ages reported that they had less difficulty concentrating and felt less sleepy during the day. Why? Because they'd slept better at night.

You get a bigger, stronger, happier, and healthier brain through exercise, too. Working out improves blood flow to and throughout your brain, stimulates hormones that promote the growth of its cells, and increases the size of the hippocampus, the part of the brain that's central to learning and memory. Exercise also helps the HPA axis—the body's central stress response system—communicate with several regions of the brain, including the limbic system, which regulates motivation and mood, and the amygdala, which controls the fight-or-flight response. Science shows that levels of anxiety, depression, and stress go down with exercise both in the long and short term. You begin to be less reactive, more thoughtful, and more able to work through the countless issues—big, small, positive, and negative—that bombard you day after day.

As you become mentally stronger, you are better able to implement and carry out a routine. In turn, this predictable structure gives you more mental strength. It's all circular. With structure, you have more freedom, and that's not just a gift of time. You suddenly develop freedom of movement and action, and don't feel trapped by a situation that's either beyond your control or bigger than you ever expected.

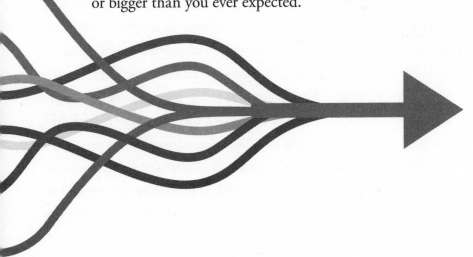

"I joined my high school's volleyball team after my mom died," Audrey told me. "I'd always liked playing, but I hadn't taken it seriously as a sport. When I suddenly had to cook dinner, clean the house, and shop for our family—just like my mom had always done—I needed some structure for myself. I needed the freedom of self-expression that came with a predictable, yet exciting, workout."

Finding exercise helped Audrey when she filled the role of a mother after her mom died, and when she became a mother to her own children. When her young children screamed at each other or threw food at the dinner table—and she didn't have a mom to call for advice—she felt in control because she'd worked out that day. Her mind worked better, she'd slept more comfortably, her self-esteem was up, her stress response was down, and she'd had something that day that was all her own.

When many of us were quarantined inside our homes during the COVID-19 pandemic, unable to wrap our brains around the uncertainty of what was happening in the world or when our lives would return to "normal"—if there *would* be a "normal" again—we still had the power to move our bodies. I've heard from lots of people that exercise was the ticket to getting through those challenging times. We could act against that mental and physical paralysis. For thirty minutes a day, five days a week, the chaos of the pandemic was not bigger or stronger than us.

We are not powerless in the face of challenges. We possess the tools to gain mental strength, control, and clarity right inside our own bodies. Exercise can help grow our brains and improve our sleep, giving us the ability to fight the physical and mental battles that face us every single day. Movement creates growth, and growth creates strength and power.

Where There's a Will, There's a Way

I'm going to draw a hard line here. When it comes to fitting exercise into your routine, there really is no excuse to skip it. Just as drinking half your body weight in water is essential to your physical and mental well-being, and you *must* do it every single day, scheduling exercise is critical. Sure, there may be a day here and there where you can't find the time, or you might have an injury or an illness that prevents you from working out for a few weeks, but the permission slips stop there. You must be deliberate about carving out time in your day and your week, and you must consciously execute those plans.

There are several different ways to go about doing this. The first is to work out at the same time every day. When I was pregnant with my twins, I didn't feel up to exercise first thing in the morning like I usually had, so I worked out at 5:30 p.m. during the work week and took the weekends off. I never scheduled meetings after 5, I planned meals ahead of time so that I didn't have to do any food prep between 5 and 6, and I made sure in advance that I always had childcare or that my children were occupied. Sometimes I just brought them in the room with me to work out. Knowing that it was a regular part of my schedule—as set in stone as dinner time and bedtime—I was able to do my

MOVE FORWARD EVERY DAY

Whenever possible, I recommend exercising first thing in the morning on an empty stomach. Not only does vigorous exercise wake you up, it's also easier to prioritize before your busy day begins or something unexpected totally derails your schedule.

When you work out with no food in your belly, your body turns to its stored fat reserves, burning as much as 20 percent more fat than it would if you'd consumed a healthy breakfast. Obviously, this has benefits in terms of increasing your lean body mass, but I've found that exercising with nothing solid in my belly is easier. I feel lighter and looser, with more of my body's energy going to my muscles and heart rather than to the food working its way slowly through my digestive system.

Some people complain that without something in their bellies they hit a wall mid-workout. If that's the case for you, try upping your liquid intake before and during your workout. Or make a twelve-ounce smoothie or green juice and drink three ounces of it before you get going. You might be surprised at how much more energy that small amount of liquid gives you.

prenatal workout all but a few times during my pregnancy, and those missed times were only because of severe nausea and vomiting. My body expected exercise, and my day flowed around it so much that I almost never found an excuse to skip it.

A second way to plan is to figure out your workout schedule at the beginning of the week, as a man named Kurt did a few months after we met. After Kurt and his wife welcomed two children in two years, Kurt became his family's primary caregiver. His job as an actor had more flexibility than his wife's job with the city government—which often required her to travel, go to late dinners, or, during an emergency like a blizzard, work all night—so he hired babysitters, cared for the children when he wasn't working, and prepared all the meals. With an irregular schedule—some days Kurt had work and other days he didn't—he found it difficult to be consistent about exercise. He became reactive with his time and promised himself he'd work out when his children went down for naps or after they went to bed at night. The problem was that some days they skipped their naps and other days he was exhausted by the time they fell asleep. He told himself he'd go to the gym after auditions, but some days his auditions would run late, and he'd have to rush home to relieve the babysitter.

When I met him, Kurt was about twenty pounds overweight with a puffy face and dark circles under his eyes.

"You should have seen me before the children," Kurt told me. "I was ripped. I went to the gym at least five times a week."

"How often do you work out now?" I asked.

"If I'm lucky, once a week. I used to go whenever I felt like it, but now, between my children's schedules and my auditions, I have no time. I have no choice but to skip it."

Kurt didn't have much flexibility in his schedule anymore, so he couldn't pick up and head to the gym at a moment's notice like he used to. He equated his inability to fly by the seat of his pants with a loss of freedom. An abundance of time and complete freedom are not really the same thing, though. As I've said a thousand times, it's *structure* that creates freedom.

What Kurt needed to do was to block out time in his calendar at the beginning of the week—or even sooner—and schedule those hour-long increments with his wife and babysitter. The truth was that the only thing standing between Kurt and walking to the gym or the park down the street with a dedicated workout space was that he hadn't planned ahead. He needed to *prioritize* scheduling that time. On top of that, he needed to get creative.

"Are there any neighbors who have children your age?" I asked him once.

"Yeah, my neighbors down the hall have twins."

There was no reason Kurt couldn't ask them to trade off childcare duties. They could take his children one day a week for an hour, then he could do the same the next day. Instead of throwing his hands up at his loss of flexibility, he could expand his social circle and help out a friend at the same time he was helping himself. In addition, he could get a jogging stroller (yes, they make them with two seats), join a gym with a daycare center, or regularly wake up a half hour earlier and dash outside for a quick jog. Working out didn't begin and end at the gym or the park. He had options, and he just needed to make exercise nonnegotiable.

Where there's a will, there's a way. And where there's a schedule, you can lock in all the many things that will help you move forward every day. With exercise, taking control of your schedule allows you to take control of your life.

MOVE FORWARD EVERY DAY

If you've been inactive much of your life, the thought of starting an exercise routine can be terrifying. Thirty minutes of sweating and aching muscles sounds awful and multiplying that pain times five sounds even worse. One of the mottoes I adopted after a mentor shared it with me is that you should "strive for progress, not perfection." The effort you make in one twenty-four-hour period is what counts as you gradually build toward a fitness program that works for you. Even if you start by jogging in place for five minutes, that's progress. A fifteen-minute walk or a few slow laps in a pool are great, and one supported pushup on your knees is amazing. The positive benefits of that exercise will flow over to the next day, when it's possible you'll be able to do more. There's no such thing as immediate perfection. Progress, however, *is* immediate, and on top of that, it's quantifiable.

10.

Stress Less

High stress means higher cortisol levels, which creates cellular damage.

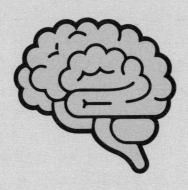

To the outside world, Rosie looked like a poster child for stress. She had two jobs, an autistic ten-year-old son, and a mother-in-law with Alzheimer's disease living with her and her husband in a cramped, two-bedroom apartment. She woke up at 5:15 a.m. to clean her kitchen, pack lunches, do a quick online workout, and fold the mountains of laundry that accumulated over the week. If he wasn't up already, she woke her son at 6:30 so he could catch the school bus at 7:15. After she kissed him goodbye, she rushed to the subway, rode an hour downtown, and was at her job at a doctor's office by 8:15. The first patients arrived at 8:30, and she was on her feet all day till 4:30, when she punched out.

She was back on the subway before 5, standing back-to-back with other rush-hour commuters so she could pick up her son from after-school an hour later. Home by 6, she waited on the stoop for her mother-in-law to arrive by bus from the care facility she went to during the day, and then she carefully helped her down the bus steps and up to their second-floor walkup.

Rosie's husband always made dinner. He was an excellent cook, so everyone sat down at the table happy to spend time together and excited to try out whatever new recipe or delicious staple he'd whipped up. Dinner was never rushed. The family talked about their days, listened to each other, and laughed. Then they moved to the small living room by 7 p.m. to watch TV.

That's when Rosie checked her emails again and started her second job. She sold cosmetics through a multilevel marketing company, and she loved the feeling of empowerment and connectivity that selling products to her circle of friends gave her. The job also earned her an extra $10,000 a year. She'd originally intended for this to be "her" money—something she could use for shopping or that rare vacation she and her husband used to take back when her mother-in-law could watch her son—but now it went to her family.

"They need it more than me," she once told me. "I can manage on my own. My mother-in-law and son require expensive programs to get the care that makes their lives better."

"Do you resent that?" I asked.

"No," she answered. "I love my family and want the best for them. I love my jobs, too, so working isn't really about the money."

Rosie was busy from the moment she got up until she crawled into bed at 10 p.m. Even the middle of the night could be demanding because her mother-in-law sometimes woke up with nightmares and wandered around the house. Yet Rosie's life wasn't chaotic, and she rarely felt the effects of what could have been a constant state of stress. She was doing *something* to make her life a success, and she was working against forces that could have pushed her body into hormonal turmoil and her mind into a place where she couldn't make good decisions or move forward.

The more I got to know her, the more I realized that Rosie wasn't doing anything that all of us can't do. I'll describe it soon. Most of us—me included—wake up early and are bombarded by pressures all day, every day. We have demanding jobs, sick relatives, screaming babies, and little to no me-time. We face trolls on social media, horrible commutes, and global pandemics. But there are ways to deal with stress that make life not just bearable, but enjoyable. How we view and process stress allows us to feel a real sense of control over our days, and with that self-mastery, we can move forward.

MOVE FORWARD EVERY DAY

While there are many valuable techniques that can lower your stress, I want to share with you a few of my stress-reducing tricks from the standpoint of health education.

- When you leave the house, always pack a lunch box. You can avoid so many stressful moments (often brought on by hunger) when you have the right food at the right time. My husband and I love lunch boxes with built-in icepacks, which are easy to find online.

- Don't ever go to bed angry or upset with your friend, spouse, or partner. Letting go of anger for a night doesn't mean you're avoiding or denying a difficult subject or conversation. Instead, you're allowing yourself to

Stress Is Karma

There are a multitude of approaches and changes you can make in your life to ward off or deal with stress, including losing weight, practicing yoga, painting, meditating, sleeping more, trying hypnosis or acupuncture, exercising, getting a dog, or hugging your spouse. I'm not going to tell you what's going to serve you best. Everyone is different, and while running outdoors and cooking are what make me feel happy, they may not work for you.

have a night of restorative sleep that will allow you to deal with the issue properly the next day. You can always say to the other person, "I love you, and I have been angry at you, but I'm not at this moment. I hope you can get some sleep, and we'll talk about this tomorrow."

• Check your to-do list a few hours before you turn in for the night so you don't get in bed convinced you've forgotten to do something or feel overwhelmed about how much you have to do the next day. Stress and sleeplessness are strongly connected, and if you come to peace with your to-do list well before bedtime, you will have time to wind down.

Besides, my approach to lessening the stress in your life has never been about adding something that takes real time and effort to your to-do list. This chapter is not about cultivating interests or finding outlets. I want to address how to change your thinking, your approach to others, and the way you order and structure your life. These broad-stroke practices will allow you to *act* through micro systems that will change the macro landscape of your life.

Let's first look at what was happening with Rosie.

Rosie's body sometimes switched into overdrive. Her day was scheduled almost down to the minute, so if her son missed the bus or her train stalled in a tunnel, she'd be late to work, and that would throw all her best-laid plans into chaos. Her body would then sound alarms. Her hypothalamus, a small region at the base of her brain, would send a signal to her adrenal glands—triangular-shaped masses located right on top of her kidneys—to release stress hormones. Adrenaline, the first of these, would flood her system, elevating her heart rate and blood pressure and increasing her energy levels. The second, cortisol, would help raise her blood-sugar levels, giving her brain and body a ready supply of glucose to fuel her as she ran toward the subway or as she calculated whether or not she should take a taxi instead. Adrenaline and cortisol would allow her to react fast and, in stressful moments, they would feel energizing and motivating, as if she had superhuman powers and could get to work on time no matter what was trying to stop her.

But only in extreme situations like these did Rosie reach this fight-or-flight state triggered by her stress hormones. When her son had an autistic meltdown in a place where he felt overwhelmed, like a crowded Target or an amusement park, she stayed as calm as possible. When her mother-in-law dropped a stack of dishes she was attempting to put away—despite the fact that Rosie had *insisted* she was too unsteady on her feet to help in the kitchen—she didn't burst into tears or run out of the house and to her neighborhood bar for a drink. She kept her stress hormones in check and prevented herself from devolving into a chronic state of stress, which would have increased her chances of developing heart disease or high blood pressure, having a stroke, or becoming obese. High cortisol and adrenaline levels can cause sleeplessness, decreased energy, and overall fatigue, but she avoided those problems. Rosie felt deeply sad sometimes, but she didn't battle the mental health challenges that plague a lot of chronically stressed people, including depression and anxiety. As I got to know Rosie, I realized that she was unconsciously doing something that my mom—a true optimist if I've ever met one—has been telling me to do since I was a child.

"MaryRuth," my mom said, "everything you feel is valid, and you should not be ashamed of your emotions. But you do not have to let your body get so upset. If you let that stress make you out of control, it's just going to bounce right back to you."

Put another way, stress is like karma. Whatever you put out there is going to return to you—in a similar or worse form—in the future.

We are all part of the collective, bound together by natural law, the order of the universe, and the fact that we live on this planet together and draw from its ecosystem. Very, very few of us live alone in the jungle or woods, completely detached from modern society. We're in this life together, and our actions affect everyone around us. If someone cuts me off in traffic and I roll down my window to yell at them, that road rage is going to make that driver tense and upset. That person might scream at me, speed up their car, or swerve into the other lane and cause an accident. If I can't restrain myself when I get bad news about a business project, and I send an angry or accusatory email to my employees, some of them may start to feel unmotivated or on edge. Those negative emotions might make them less productive, making my job harder. And if Rosie screamed at her son for refusing to put his shoes on before they walked out of their apartment in the morning, he might start to fumble with the laces and break out in tears. He'd miss his bus, Rosie would be late to work, and absolutely everything would be more stressful in their lives.

There should be no disconnect between the way you treat people and the way you want to be treated. I don't say this from any moral or religious stance, either. I'm being purely practical. If you act with compassion toward difficult people, they're more likely to be normal and sane with you. And if you want to have less stress in your life, you should put less stress out into the world.

We've all met people who are like dark clouds. These individuals walk into a room with a scowl on their faces and begin to say cutting, biting remarks to everyone in their path. Or maybe they don't say anything, they just cast negative thoughts, changing the quantum energy of what was otherwise a happy spot. I'm not telling you that you can't have a bad day, but you simply can't deny that your thoughts and your actions have a ripple effect that doesn't just impact others. They also affect *you*. Think of your actions like a motorboat that's cutting fast through a big, peaceful lake. The wake that boat leaves rocks the other boats back and forth, knocks people on water skis and paddleboards into the water, and causes waves on the shore. When your boat circles back around, it hits that wake again, making your path forward choppy and turbulent.

What we're going for is the energy balance we talked about in action six. The happiest, most directed people in the world are those whose internal energy matches or balances the external energy that surrounds them and that they share with others. While I don't think you can stop a raging house fire just by putting out good energy, I'm sure you can deal with that horrible situation in a much more controlled manner—and get better results—if you're not getting more upset than is actually warranted.

Ever heard of the butterfly effect? This is similar. The butterfly effect proposes that something as small as the ripple of a butterfly's wings can cause quantum changes in the world's energy balance and eventually lead to catastrophic effects like a hurricane. Try not to be that butterfly. The payback, karma, return (or whatever you choose to call it) you'll see coming from the outside world will be much more stable if you attempt to stress less. Bridging the disconnect between the exter- nal and the internal is *entirely* within your power.

MOVE FORWARD EVERY DAY

How many of you have faced a deadline and experienced a rush of cortisol that's pushed you to stay up till the wee hours and work harder than you normally do? Pretty much all of us. Now, faced with that same deadline, how many of you have also rushed to the office snack machine or dug through the pantry looking for a bag of chips or a box of donuts? My guess is that's all of you, too. Elevated cortisol levels and cravings go hand in hand. Cortisol causes your blood sugar to spike fast so you can have a ready supply of energy, but then it plummets just as quickly. When your blood sugar becomes dramatically lower than it was before, your body screams for you to eat—especially carbs and sugary snacks.

If cortisol levels remain chronically high and you don't curb your snack habit, you're more likely to put on weight in your belly rather than other areas of your body. We have more cortisol receptors in the fat on our midsection than we do on other fatty areas, so, if you're stressed, the pounds you put on will land on your stomach first.

That's the principle Rosie worked from. Rosie spent the first three years of her son's life struggling to get a diagnosis for him. When he began screaming and melting down after she turned on the vacuum and when she cut his sandwiches in squares rather than diagonals, her head spun and her pulse raced. She *knew* something was wrong, and she felt out of control because no one could tell her exactly what it was. But then she took a deep breath and did whatever she needed to in order to think straight and stop her body from being so upset. Faced with a helpless person who was feeling more turmoil—not to mention cortisol and adrenaline—than she was, she chose calm over chaos. The more she trained herself to do this, the easier it became. Soon, her family picked up on her positive vibes, and they calmed down, too. The external energy inside their small apartment began to match each person's internal energy—and that had all started because Rosie took control and acted.

Take Stock of Yourself

When I worked as a certified health educator, many of my clients were uber successful CEOs, heads of nonprofits, business owners, and sales professionals who'd built their careers from nothing. Yes, there were a few who'd inherited money or gotten a foot in the door from social connections, but most were people who'd risked everything to start careers with little or no outside help. I relate so much to people like this because I've been there myself. Every penny I made after I started my company went toward paying off our personal debt rather than back into my company, so nothing went to waste. To be certain that my money was spent properly and that everything was accounted for, I made spreadsheets and lists and backed up my documents multiple times. I printed out every email and filed them away in labeled folders, with all the papers facing the same direction. Not a single conversation—in-person, on the phone, or via email, text, or social media—was unaccounted for. I knew how thin my margins were and how every choice had a financial consequence, so I took stock of everything and worked hard on a daily basis.

Without fail, all my clients who'd created their dream careers from scratch had done the same. Scrutinizing every decision and every action made a great deal of sense to them, so when I told them to look through their refrigerator every morning to pave the way for making healthier food choices, not a single one of them had a problem doing it. In fact, it seemed so logical that many wondered why they hadn't done it sooner. When they sat down to work, they had no issue determining where their business had fallen short the day, week, month, or year before, how they could improve, and what it would take to catapult their business model into the future. Success came through organization and seizing control promised to help them put their careers on comfortable and smooth autopilot.

If you want to reduce stress in your life and put your mind and body on autopilot, you should be doing the exact same thing for yourself. Once a week—if not more—sit down and take stock of yourself in the same way you account for the items on your work to-do list, your company's five-year plan, and the food in your refrigerator. Get out a pen and paper, voice recorder, or any other note-taking method, and take a good, hard look at yourself.

Start with the big picture by thinking about these kinds of questions: *Last week didn't go as well as I wanted it to go. Why? Where did I just give up? What kind of stress smacked me in the face because of that?* At first, you might not be able to pinpoint exactly where things went wrong or how your behavior played into it, but you might be able to next week. Simply starting the process of self-examination transfers accountability and power back to you.

Your list should include urgent, stressful issues and items that aren't urgent yet still cause you to worry. For example, you might hate mammograms because your mom had breast cancer, but your annual mammogram needs to happen this month, and you still haven't scheduled it. That's urgent, so write it down. Your daughter is graduating from high school in a year and you really want to do something special for her, like take a family vacation or throw a big party, but planning events is not your strong suit and thinking about it stresses you out. That's not really urgent but you should still write it down.

If you like, you can work your inventory into a checklist, so you can tally what you've done and haven't done over the week. Checking off an accomplishment will feel like a victory. If you have to return to an issue or problem the following week, you'll have it right there, ready to tackle when the time is right.

This is not a list of resolutions, so don't add things like "I want to read more" unless the fact that you haven't read a book in a year makes you feel anxious. Don't worry about how seemingly insignificant in the scheme of your life your hot-button concerns are. If something causes you any amount of stress, it's worth taking stock of. These minute bits of tension are the things that can stop you in your tracks, paralyzing you for a few seconds or minutes and elevating your cortisol and adrenaline. That tension adds up and causes a negative emotional reaction. You might become angry or resentful about your place in life, or you might try to run away from the problem. Unfortunately, problems don't just go away. Your poorly functioning dishwasher that causes you to handwash everything placed on the top rack isn't going to magically fix itself. It's been broken for six months, and you've spent ten minutes every morning gritting your teeth as you handwashed your dishes. After a year, that's thirty hours of stressful lost time you will never get back.

Don't be afraid to include issues over which you have no control. Rosie's list included the uncertainty of how her mother-in-law's illness would progress and how it would play out in the space of their home. Would she wander away from home one day and go missing, like many people with Alzheimer's do? Would her needs grow beyond what Rosie and her husband could offer her? Just having those broad questions on her list week after week showed Rosie that she and her husband needed to discuss them, comfort each other, keep the dialogue open, prepare, and act on what they could. Planning could prevent their bodies from being reactive. Writing problems down made them seem less insurmountable and daunting. She could account for them. She could name them. And, someday, she could act on them and try to change them.

I'm going to share my honest opinion here: refusing to take stock of where you're falling behind in your life is more than just a bad habit. It is procrastination and a form of laziness. If you want long-term fulfillment, you need to take real, serious responsibility and own up to the fact that procrastination and laziness are going to cause stress and prevent you from taking the small actions that will create a momentum that moves you forward toward happiness.

Laziness is *not* a character flaw, though, and you're not a bad person if you struggle to tackle things you don't really feel like doing. I know that fighting against the idleness that slows us down can be incredibly hard work. It can also be deeply personal and may brush up against real emotional trauma, forcing us to face secrets that are painful to deal with. The financial debt my mom and I fell into in the late 2010s was mortifying to me. The girls I grew up with had big, fancy weddings, while we couldn't afford a cake and my $200 engagement ring left a rash on my finger. I know having a low-cost wedding isn't the end of the world, but I was so embarrassed about my financial situation that I didn't talk to anyone about it except a few people who I was certain wouldn't judge me. You may be hiding the fact that you're gay from your parents. Or maybe you have an incurable, yet treatable, STD and feel sick about the prospect of telling the guy you just started dating. These secrets could be smaller: you planned to drink less than ten drinks a week, yet you drank twelve and hid the two extra beer bottles from your husband. You forgot to order your mom flowers for Mother's Day, and you don't want to tell your brother, who asked you to do it. Regardless of whether

MOVE FORWARD EVERY DAY

I want to be clear that while laziness can be depressing, depression and laziness are two very different things. Depression is not a choice, and when you're suffering from it you may not even notice the pile of filthy clothes you left on your bedroom floor or the fact that you haven't changed your sheets in three weeks. When you're lazy, you're making a choice to leave your clothes on the ground or sleep on dirty sheets. Depression renders you unable to act. If you suffer from it, you need to seek professional help. The cure for laziness is entirely within your power, and you can turn it around by creating structure and accounting for yourself and your actions. The cure for depression lies in seeking help from a professional.

you can confide in anyone, you have to be honest with yourself. If you refuse to take stock of where you are in your life—or, on a smaller scale, in your week—that stress will eat you up. The person you are on the inside won't match what you're trying to project to the outside world, and, once again, your external and internal energy will be out of whack. That causes stress and pain.

Creating a predictable routine for yourself can be the perfect antidote to laziness and the energy imbalance that plagues so many of us. Setting aside one time a week—or more if you feel it's necessary—to take stock of yourself and where you want to be in your life helps you regain tons of power. Stress is a force that works against our forward momentum every day, and the way to overcome it is to take control and act. Relaxing or running away for a few days to take a vacation are great and can be tremendously helpful in the short term, but they just postpone the inevitable. Relaxation as a way of life isn't stress relief; it *causes* unnecessary stress. However, making a reasonable system to take stock of yourself every week will allow you to act, and that will help you feel more in control of your life and, ultimately, happier.

Stop Procrastinating and Make Your Life Easier

If you think that most of your life is stressful and you're living out that stress through your thoughts and actions, you need to do everything in your power, leaving no stone unturned, to try to make it better. Procrastinating does more than get you nowhere. It moves you backward rather than forward every day.

When your cortisol levels are persistently high, the neurons in your *prefrontal cortex*—the part of the brain responsible for planning, decision-making, and behavior—begin to die. When your prefrontal cortex can't be as active as it once was, your judgment becomes skewed, and you may struggle with planning and making good decisions. On top of that, high cortisol levels suppress activity in your *hippocampus*—the part of your brain involved in learning and memory—and decrease serotonin. Without enough of your happiness hormone, you'll become angrier, sadder, and more aggressive. When you're easily frustrated, it's harder for you to do the things that make life worth living and that move you ahead. Chronic stress causes a vicious playback loop, but the good news is that you can break it by not procrastinating and by doing the things that make your life easier.

After you take stock of yourself, look at your list. What can you tackle today? What's most urgent? What's going to require the least amount of energy but deliver the greatest results? I'm sure you're not going to be able to get to all the items on your list immediately, but doing just one small action will give you power and will create momentum and desire to do *another* action.

MOVE FORWARD EVERY DAY

Relationships—especially marriages and partnerships—are often the greatest cause of stress in our lives. Couples clash about all kinds of things, from money to how to discipline children to whether to sell the house. If one person doesn't assume their expected role within the family for whatever reason (illness, depression, a new job, or a betrayal such as an affair), it's incredibly stressful for everyone they're close to. A great deal rides on two people working together, and when one person falls short, fights can follow. And they can be *huge*.

A couple I'm close friends with just spent a few months in couples' therapy because they both thought they were arguing too much about money. I'm happy to say their marriage came

For example, a few months ago, my house had one smoke detector that went off in the middle of the night. This happened about once a month, and it woke us up and forced me to stumble around half asleep looking for a step stool so I could climb up and turn it off. The smoke detector was hardwired rather than battery powered, so it took time to turn it off and, while it beeped and beeped and beeped, I'd become so frustrated that it would be almost impossible to fall back asleep afterward.

I fixed the smoke detector three times and each time I convinced myself I'd found the solution. But since I have no expertise

out of therapy stronger and it was, in part, due to some advice their therapist gave them.

"In any fight," the therapist said, "one person is more upset than the other. It's the responsibility of the person who's less triggered to do whatever they need to do to end the argument."

Think about that next time you're in an argument. Are you less upset than your business partner or husband? Acknowledge it to yourself. Then begin to listen, and don't be reactive. Recognize the other's person's complaints and even say to them, "I'm less upset than you, so I'm not going to escalate this situation." Radiating that calm control will have a ripple effect, and chances are you'll begin to solve your problems sooner rather than later.

whatsoever as far as electrical wiring goes, a few weeks later, the smoke detector started beeping again.

It may sound silly, but the fear of the smoke detector going off in the middle of the night really put me on edge, especially because I value sleep so much. Each time I walked under it, I'd start to doubt whether I'd really fixed it. When I lay in bed at night, I'd start to worry. *Is it going to go off again? Where did I leave the step stool?* Even if that stress delayed me falling asleep by two minutes, those were two minutes that counted in the scheme of my life.

After the smoke detector went off in the middle of the night a fourth time, I set aside a three-hour block of time on a weekend, had my husband take my older boys to the park, and installed a new smoke alarm that actually worked. My family hasn't been jolted awake in the middle of the night for almost a year, and I feel *so much better.* When I look at that smoke detector, I can tell myself: *I will never be the effect again. I will only be the cause.* That sense of accomplishment may seem small, but, in that moment, it's super empowering.

Don't procrastinate on taking action to make your life easier in whatever way you can. If there's a person on Facebook or Twitter or Instagram whose posts irritate you so much that you stop what you're working on, ignore your loved ones, and waste three minutes of your life typing an angry response that you regret later, it's time you block that person. If this issue keeps cropping up for you, get off these sites entirely. There is absolutely no need for you to add that unnecessary stress to your life.

The goal is to chip away at the stressful emotional blocks in your life, big and small. Write down all the things that bother you and stop you in your tracks every day, and then force yourself to tackle them. When you do, I promise you'll find you have greater momentum in your life. Soon, it'll be like you're driving down a road with no traffic or speed bumps, and one green light followed by another. Every time a red light comes, instead of procrastinating, you'll know what to do right away.

11.

Think Positively

Use positive thoughts
to imbue your day with gratitude.

I've always been results-oriented and hands-on, so when I developed my program in 2013, the actions that were most like how I lived my life were by far the easiest for me to wrap my brain around. I might be stuck in a bad situation and think, *Okay, maybe I can't fix this problem today, but if I sleep more, chew my food till it's liquid, and organize my refrigerator, I can get up enough energy to figure out what steps to take.* These very tangible actions put me in my comfort zone, set me on a forward path, and gave me a real sense of accomplishment. They allowed me to feel inspired, powerful, and optimistic, and they validated my paradigm of wellness and functionality. To me, it was pretty simple: you can rebuild from suffering or negativity by acting in practical ways, and you can fill up your scorecard in life just by doing things that deliver immediate mental and physical benefits.

Imagine my surprise when I fell in love with someone whose approach to living life is almost completely abstract. To my husband, David, moving forward in life has always been about embracing the spiritual and searching for your larger purpose. Instead of latching on to small, concrete actions that add up to large-scale personal change, he chooses to look at the big picture, visualizing a larger transformation that doesn't necessarily depend on concrete physical or emotional outcomes. He asks the intangible questions; I make lists. When we met, he'd taken a vow of poverty so he could help bring spirituality to the world; I'd taken a job as a Manhattan real estate agent to help us pay our rent. He now teaches spirituality; I tell people to take their vitamins every day.

David and I were born on the same day in the same year—exactly two hours and twenty-four minutes apart—so maybe we were just meant to be. Our relationship also has a thousand wonderful complexities, so I don't mean to simplify it. David *is* very logical, and when I left my real estate job to work as a certified health educator—even though it meant doing free consultations at first, and even though we had nothing in our checking account and a lot of debt—David told me he loved me and supported my dreams but that I was completely crazy. But the reality is that, just like me and David, most people are basically one or the other: spiritual and feeling or practical and action oriented. It could be that you're born a certain way, or it might be that your parents drilled your beliefs and practices into you at an early age. It really doesn't matter.

What *does* matter is this: those of you out there who struggle with existential concepts like positivity do not need to worry. The tangible, small actions you take to move your life forward blend seamlessly into larger discussions of energy, spirituality, and the soul. Yes, it's hard, time-consuming, sometimes scary work to embrace the spiritual, but seeing these broad, existential concepts is vital to your life. The great news is that doing micro actions makes it much easier, and, in this action, I'll give you concrete ways to harness the power of your mind to think more positively.

Sometimes my concepts will be theoretical, but I will back them up with examples that practical people can use and enjoy.

This action is not "101 Easy Ways to Be Happy." I wrote this book in 2020, a year when we faced a pandemic and social crisis and change that felt so unreal that it might as well have been from a movie. The year 2020 stretched my brain into some pretty new places and taught me that there are no quick fixes to moving your life—and the world—in a positive direction. Instead, we need to dig deep within our minds, bodies, and spirits and take personal responsibility in order to change the way we think. It's hard work, but it is necessary and *so* worth it.

Positivity Is a Choice Your Mind Makes

No one is born a pessimist. Babies innately know to reach out for others, looking for comfort, and, as they grow, they constantly strive to do better, get stronger, and learn more in order to bolster their happiness. Over time, though, the disappointments and traumas of everyday life may shift people's minds from optimism to pessimism. Life can wear you down, causing you to think about the bad things more than the good. You don't have to be stuck in this place. Positivity can be learned, and you can practice making it part of your life.

My husband and I talk a lot about why we chose to start a family, especially one with four children spaced less than four years apart. Having children forces you to accept incredible stress, including money pressures, hard decisions about whose career

MOVE FORWARD EVERY DAY

Sometimes when we're forced to tackle abstract or large-scale issues in life, the only way to drum up the courage or strength to do it is to act in *any* kind of small way. It doesn't matter if you're following a program. Just do *something*. Engage in some type of small action that will allow the process of momentum to begin moving you forward.

For example, some therapists say that if you're feeling depressed, you should try to clean your house. The issue isn't that a messy home can add to your feelings of hopelessness (though it can). The fact is that doing something tangible gives you a sense of self-control and empowerment, which in turn gives you purpose and guides you just the tiniest bit ahead.

comes first and who handles the chores, loss of sleep and personal space, and a complete surrender of what you feel is "right" or "normal." I used to think that certain children would never throw tantrums. Now I know that children don't follow rules all the time; they can be messy, chaotic, and a lot of hard work.

So why would a person choose to have children? Many want to be part of something bigger than themselves or have a larger purpose. Faced with the negativity and stress in the world, a lot of people want to believe there is something hopeful out there. The innocence of a new life could be the thing that moves their lives and the world in a positive direction.

Whether or not to start a family isn't my point, though. What I'm saying is that we all have a purpose in life, and it's a positive, hopeful objective that's entirely up to us to pursue. We can ignore our purpose and choose negativity if we want, but I don't believe that's the place your mind wants to be. There is natural law and order to the world, and it teaches us to grow, strive for something better, and transform negativity into positivity. It's entirely up to your incredibly powerful mind to follow through on that choice.

Let's look at an example. Imagine that you have two young children, and you and your husband decide to get a divorce. You get primary custody of the children, which means you're doing most of the daily hard work like helping them with their homework, pushing them out the door every day for school, organizing playdates and activities, and telling them to clean up their rooms.

Every other weekend, your ex and your ex's beautiful, younger girlfriend come over in their fancy sports car. Your children are *so* excited because their dad takes them to Disneyland and water parks on the weekend. They get all the vegan ice cream they want and don't have to go to bed till midnight. Weekends with "Disneyland Dad," as your friends call him, are so fun that your children complain when they come home on Sunday—right after they've dumped a load of dirty laundry on your bedroom floor. As you think about your ex and his beautiful girlfriend, you resent him. You're hurt and negative, have too much laundry and too many chores, and haven't had a decent date in ages.

Now, imagine your elderly mom who lives out of town calls to tell you she's going to the hospital for emergency surgery. You have to spend $1,000 you don't have on a flight to see her and, for three days, you eat hospital food, sleep in a chair, and talk to doctors about your mom's precarious health. You think about how much your mom means to you and how worried about her you are, and you start to miss all the mundane things you do with your children. Suddenly, the laundry doesn't seem so bad and your old minivan reminds you of the songs you and your children sing while you blast music on the way to school. And thank God for Disneyland Dad! He was right there to take your children when you dashed out of town, and not for a second have you worried about your children's happiness or whether they're well taken care of. Disneyland Dad and his girlfriend are right there to make it all better.

Between these two situations, nothing about your ex-husband or children changed. You were simply in a different place in life and you chose to think about your ex more positively. *All* the power was in your mind because positivity is a mindset over which we have complete control. We can expand our lens, shift our perspective, and discover a new way to see the world.

Choose Not to Be a Victim

Sometimes choosing to think positively is not just about making a mental shift, it's about backing up that mental choice with actions.

My brother, Daniel, was a starting pitcher of his varsity high school baseball team. On April 8, 2004, I drove home from Fairfield University in Connecticut to the town we lived in for Easter break. It was a Thursday, and Daniel always had baseball games on Thursday nights.

I was in the crowd watching Daniel's team play and, while I can't recall if they won or lost, I remember being so proud of my brother. He was tall like me, and when he wound up and threw the ball his limbs looked strong and steady. My little brother was confident and fully in control. He was the leader of a team he loved more than almost anything, and I'm not sure I'd seen him that happy in a long time.

Daniel didn't look sick. In fact, he really wasn't, at least on the surface. But inside, his heart's inner walls had grown thick and hard and his heart was twice its normal weight. Daniel had been born with the genetic heart disease hypertrophic cardiomyopathy, and it had developed without any visible signs or warnings. The day after his baseball game, Daniel had tried some cocaine a younger female classmate gave him late Friday night and his heart couldn't take it. My mom found him dead the next morning.

His friends told us it was the first time Daniel had tried cocaine, and it is worth noting that only a small amount of it was in his system. He did not overdose. It doesn't make a difference, though, because the medical doctors (who performed the autopsy) said that a single dose of over-the-counter cold medicine could have stopped his diseased heart. But in the midst of our unbearable grief, my mom and I were faced with a difficult decision. There's a law in New Jersey that states that if person is given drugs by someone and then dies, the supplier is held liable for their role in the death. There is strict liability for drug-induced deaths.

A short criminal investigation determined who'd given my brother the cocaine, and my mom and I had to make a choice. Would we pursue a case or not? We agonized, discussed, listed the pros and cons, and attempted to predict how we'd feel in months or years. Projecting grief's path is useless, of course, because it pivots almost daily. Finally, we decided not to go after the classmate who'd given Daniel the cocaine. We reasoned that while one person's life had ended, another person didn't have to be destroyed on top of it. She'd been careless, selfish, and shortsighted, but her mistake was probably going to eat away at her for the rest of her life. We didn't have to feel like victims, too. Life had been unspeakably hard for me and my mom, but we were going to rise above it.

I understand how someone might disagree with our decision, believing that people should be held accountable for their actions. But for me and my mom, choosing to move forward was a positive action that put our hearts and minds in a stronger place. We already felt like casualties of a genetic fluke and one careless decision, but we didn't want to feed into that chaos by casting ourselves into the role of victims. Looking for satisfaction or closure from the wheels of the justice system as they worked against another person felt deeply negative. There was no justice in Daniel's death, and no one was going to make things better for us. We had to do the work to save ourselves.

MOVE FORWARD EVERY DAY

Your gut and your brain are linked and the foods you eat affect your thoughts and your ability to be positive. On the flip side, the quality of your thoughts influence how you digest your food. Think of your digestive tract as your second brain. When you have "butterflies in your stomach" because of something you're nervous about, it isn't just a saying. Your belly really *is* feeling the commotion caused by your thoughts.

Stress, anxiety, or negativity can affect the movement and contraction of the GI tract, so when you're upset about something, you might experience digestive upset, gas, bloating, diarrhea, or constipation. People with diagnosed GI disorders also feel pain more strongly than those without these conditions, proving that their brain is more sensitive to signals from their gut.

Pay attention to your emotions when you eat. If you begin to experience GI symptoms during tough times, don't write them off. Your belly is trying to tell you something, so seek the help or self-care you need.

Positivity is a choice backed by action. Those actions can be intensely personal and entirely specific to your situation, but the common denominator is that you *must* depend on yourself. You may be accused of being selfish, but choosing to be a victim only makes you insecure, and that is a very, very negative way to be. Resolve to be positive and move forward in whatever way is right for you. If I'd spent five years seeking "justice" for the person who gave drugs to my brother, I know I'd feel like a victim, and I know I wouldn't be where I am today in terms of happiness.

Being Positive Is Hard Work

Putting yourself into a positive position in life is not easy. The decision my mom and I made took days of soul searching, more than a few tears, and a few disagreements that could have devolved into huge fights if we hadn't been so worn out. Then, after we put the case to bed, we had to face our grief, my mom's two benign brain tumors, two benign breast tumors of my own, and our eventual financial ruin. Life has dragged us both over the coals time and time again, and sometimes I feel intense emotional pain. But the hard work to become positive is worth it at the end of the day. Every day, I take personal responsibility for my toxic internal environment and any negative internal thoughts I may have. I've done therapy, spiritual work, and my twelve actions (probably a thousand times), and when I've failed, I've started from scratch. It's labor, but it's a labor of love for myself, my family, and the person I want to be in this world.

I think a lot about a client of mine named Charlie. Charlie was a force of nature and, as a project manager who oversaw about twenty people, he never let a challenging situation at work stop him from trying to make his team function smoothly. He was the person all his friends turned to for advice because he could make smart, sensible decisions at a moment's notice. He didn't agonize over what was right or what was wrong. Instead, like the leader he was, he weighed the positives and the negatives, asked others for their feedback, and envisioned a path forward. Then, he acted.

Charlie's parents had always been a negative force in his life. His dad was a lifelong alcoholic, and he'd abandoned him, his mom, and his little sister when Charlie was fifteen. His mom,

MOVE FORWARD EVERY DAY

While it's normal to have emotional highs and lows during your day, if you're waking up every morning full of dread and anxiety, struggling to pull yourself out from under the covers, your body is trying to tell you something. Especially if you have a lot of negative energy and internally negative thoughts, sadness, and depression, even when you try as hard as possible to change your mindset, don't ignore it.

Seeking good mental health counseling from a professional is an essential first step. Another step to consider is looking at your diet. A few days or weeks before, what you ate may have caused the pH level in your cells to become more acidic.

rather than feeling relieved that he was gone and that she now had a chance to rebuild her family, chose to become a victim. She blamed her husband for the fact that she had to start her life over in her forties, go back to work, and send her children to college on one salary. "Your no-good father ruined our lives!" she always said. Then, just like the man she despised but couldn't shake off, she turned to drinking.

Charlie became hyperresponsible in the face of his mom's defeat, picking up his sister at school, making dinner, and doing all the grocery shopping on the weekend. He also made enough money mowing lawns to buy himself a car when he left for college. But a great many of us are shaped by our moms, and Charlie

While there is some research on how acidic pH levels worsen the symptoms of bipolar disorder and schizophrenia, studies of "normal" brains are limited. But in all my years working with clients, I've noticed that the more acidic your diet, the more anxiety and stress in your life. Our cells just don't want an excess of acidic foods like gluten grains, sugars, meat, and processed foods. Your diet needs to be balanced out with alkaline foods like fruits, vegetables, nuts, and seeds. On a cellular level, acidic cells create negative thoughts. Negative thoughts create negative words, and negative words create negative actions.

was no exception. He internalized all his mom's pessimism and became a big, dark cloud, especially when he drank.

"My negativity—especially when I drink—is the only thing my husband ever complains about with me," he said sadly one day.

I encouraged him to do everything in his power to feel positive about his life—even for a moment. If he was upset, he had to take a small action. If he was angry for no reason, he had to do the work. So, every morning, Charlie woke up and meditated for fifteen minutes. Three times a week, he worked out with his husband. He did regular juice cleanses, and he tried as hard as possible to do my program. He decided to start each week sending messages to his friends bright and early Monday mornings, saying something like, "You can do it! Have a great week!"

Then he quit drinking, which was probably the hardest thing he'd ever done. He'd never been a frequent drinker, but when he drank maybe twice a month, he went over the top. For one carefree night, he could dance on the table without worrying about what anyone thought of him or how many responsibilities he had at work. Unfortunately, the alcohol made him mean, negative, and thoughtless—like his mom had always been. He yelled at his husband for things he normally wouldn't, and he blamed him for anything that had gone wrong in his day.

Charlie's path to being positive wasn't perfect. Sometimes he slipped up at an office party and had a drink or two, and sometimes he spent his morning workouts mentally listing all the insignificant yet irritating things his husband did. But he *tried* to be optimistic. And the simple fact that he'd made the effort gave him a sense of self-mastery and happiness.

Pretending you're happy or that you enjoy a particular hobby doesn't force you into a positive place. If you're a square peg, you're not going to fit into a round hole. You have to be honest with yourself in all your actions. Charlie didn't work out because he thought it might make him interesting or upbeat; he actually liked the endorphin rush it gave him. He didn't send positive texts to his friends when he was having a bad day. He meditated for a few minutes, thought of something he was grateful for, and then pushed send. The external energy Charlie received from those endorphins or a nice text from a friend matched his good internal energy, and that moved his day forward in a positive direction.

100 Percent Involvement, but Detachment from the Outcome

This may not sound logical, but I believe that in order to be positive about the actions you're taking to move forward in your life, sometimes you need to imagine the worst possible outcome.

When my oldest son, Ethan, was seventeen months old and was diagnosed with moderate *hypotonia* (low muscle tone), David and I were shocked but not surprised. We'd constantly felt that hollow feeling in our guts that told us something was really wrong. Ethan had always struggled to stand up while grabbing on to his crib or a table, and he'd never been one of those babies whose hands you could hold on to while you helped him walk forward. His legs were like noodles, and he couldn't crawl, stand, or walk.

David and I wasted no time coming up with a plan, and our first step was to settle on a goal.

"I want Ethan to walk by the time he goes to preschool when he's two and a half," I said.

Ethan was seventeen months old, so that goal was just over a year away. It may sound like plenty of time to parents of children who haven't struggled to walk, but Ethan's muscle tone was so poor that I knew everything we did was going to be an uphill battle.

Then David and I played out the worst-case scenario in our heads, accepting that all our hard work might never pay off. I pictured Ethan in a wheelchair, and I thought about the changes we'd have to make to our home, the activities I wouldn't be able to enroll him in, and the challenges he'd encounter throughout his life. I saw all the scary stuff that no parent ever wants to think about, and then I told myself, *It's going to be fine. David and I love Ethan more than anything. He will always have a home and the same opportunities as his brother. He'll have the best care in the world, a place to work, and anything his little heart desires.*

I played out a terrible—yet possible—result and, guess what? It wasn't that bad. The thought of Ethan in a wheelchair didn't make me want to give up; it motivated me to work harder knowing that maybe, just maybe, we could avoid it. Imagining the worst took the pressure off all the work David, Ethan, and I had to do, and we felt empowered to move forward.

Those of you out there who are familiar with Alcoholics Anonymous might know the idea of hitting rock bottom. This is the belief that an alcoholic must reach their lowest, most desperate point before they can admit they have a problem and seek change. This bottom could be losing your children in a custody battle, killing someone in a drunk-driving accident, going to jail, or even something as minor as waking up with a really bad hangover. Charlie told me months after we first met that what prompted him to go to AA was his husband saying, "I'm afraid you're turning into your mom, and I don't want to be married to that person." Regardless, rock bottom is a precipitating event that shows a person that alcohol has made their lives unmanageable and that they have to quit.

What's transformational to some people—like Charlie—is that although seeing the worst-case scenario actually come to pass might be crushing, it's also a relief.

"When my husband suggested he might leave me someday, it was the worst thing I could imagine," Charlie said. "But then I realized I could live differently. I had the freedom to stop drinking, and that was exciting. The fact that saving my wonderful marriage was entirely up to me was very empowering."

Glimpsing the worst-case scenario opens up a world of possibilities. Sure, you know the work ahead may be grueling and the days might be long, but at least there's no dread. Being free of that paralyzing fear is such a positive position to be in, and it can motivate you through whatever you have to do, big or small.

The Power of Resilience

Resilience is a term that's thrown around any time there's a tragedy in the world, but I've found that many people don't quite understand what it means. They believe resilience is strength, but in fact it's a lot bigger and more profound than that. Resilience is the ability to grow and adapt in the face of trauma, adversity, change, or stress. It's the capacity to power through a difficult experience and come out on the other side altered, but still thriving. When you're strong, you can withstand something tough. But when you're resilient, you can overcome and move past it.

When you're resilient and face something challenging, your path won't be easy. In fact, the American Psychological Association says that, by definition, resilience goes hand-in-hand with significant emotional distress. But your catastrophes won't paralyze you or define the rest of your life. They may make you a different person in some ways, but you won't necessarily be trapped in those horrible moments forever.

Recently I read an article in *Psychology Today* that spoke volumes to me. The author, a counselor named Danielle Render Turmaud, writes that resilience has never been about bouncing back from a traumatic incident. If it were, you would return from a tragedy to the exact same place you started. You wouldn't learn anything, nor would you mature emotionally. Instead, resilient people "bounce forward." They'll still face challenges in the future because there's no such thing as "happily ever after" in life, but resilience grants you the tools to make your life happy in spite of what you endure. When you bounce forward, you have self-mastery, self-awareness, and strength. You can cope *and* you can grow, adapt, and become energized even when the stress of life pushes back on you.

I'm often reminded of what a friend of mine said about a mutual friend who'd lost her three year old in a tragic accident, then become pregnant a few months later.

"When your child dies, what choice do you have? You can either be stuck in the paralysis of that horrible death, or you can literally create a new life."

I've seen this with my own family. I watched my mother bury her husband and seventeen-year-old son, and then I watched her rebuild her life. I learned everything about the concept of moving forward every day from my mom.

There's been a great deal of scientific research about what makes a person resilient, and it has shown that genetics play a very small part. One of the most important factors is a network of close relationships, especially with those you consider your caretakers. If the individuals who raised you made you feel loved, safe, and cared for—especially during difficult times—they helped your brain develop the right way so it could manage the stress response, process bad events, and make good decisions. Essentially, good primary caregivers hand you the tools that allow you to become resilient.

One of the other big benefits of resilience is the ability to stay positive even when things are bad. In 2005, Dr. Dennis Charney, a professor of psychiatry and neuroscience from the Mount Sinai

School of Medicine in New York City, presented his findings from a study of 750 Vietnam War–veterans who'd been kept as prisoners of war for six to eight years. These men had been subjected to unspeakable torture and cruelty, but, amazingly, none of them had developed PTSD or suffered from significant bouts of depression afterward. Charney tested and interviewed these men and determined that the central factor behind their resilience was their optimism. These men hadn't necessarily had happy endings in life—they'd experienced death, illness, and other tragedies, many of which felt as painful as their imprisonment—but they hadn't fallen into helplessness. Their optimism had allowed them to bounce forward.

Dr. Barbara Fredrickson is one of the world's most well-respected scholars in the field of positive psychology and, as the director of the Positive Emotions and Psychophysiology Laboratory at the University of North Carolina, Chapel Hill, her research on the connection between positivity and resilience has been groundbreaking. One of her studies looked at a group of people who were asked to do a task, then exposed to an emotionally negative video clip. When compared to another group of people who were asked to do the same task, then watched a positive clip, the subjects who encountered positivity showed a marked decline in physical symptoms of stress, including increased heart rate and blood pressure. In short, happy thoughts can help lessen the uncomfortable physical reactions that result from a stressful situation.

Frederickson's research went on to show that when people who aren't particularly resilient are given a stressful task and told

MOVE FORWARD EVERY DAY

No matter how young your children are, they can learn to be positive. I saw an amazing story last year about a young boy named Sammy Silver who was born with a disease called *osteogenesis imperfecta*, or brittle bone disease. His bones are so fragile that, by the time he was three-and-a-half, he'd fractured forty bones and had had six surgeries. His bones could break when his parents simply changed his clothes or when he went to get his blood drawn.

Faced with something no parent ever imagines, his mom, Allison, said the most important thing for their son was to stay positive. From day one she and Sammy's dad repeated positive affirmations with him, and now he wakes up every morning with a smile on his face. He says his affirmations by himself now, repeating "I tough! I brave! I strong! I Sammy Silver!"

I do this with my own children now, and they love it. They *are* tough and brave, so why not sing it out? Even if they're motivated to think positively for just a split second, I promise it will make a difference. You'll smile, then they'll smile, and suddenly you've both put something positive into your lives.

to view it as an opportunity, their heart rates and blood pressure improve. When they're told to view the same job as a threat, heart rate and blood pressure worsen. Basically, positivity and optimism don't just help you deal with past events; they allow you to be more resilient and stronger heading into future events, too.

People with a positive outlook live on average 11 to 15 percent longer than they would if they chose negativity, and they're more likely to live past age eighty-five. That's much more time to enjoy life, reap the physical benefits of optimism, and spend time with the people you love. So, think positively: it will carry you through today, tomorrow, and beyond.

12.

Believe in a Universal Force of Goodness

It doesn't matter what you call that universal force—God, Creator—it just matters that you believe that the universe wants the best for you.

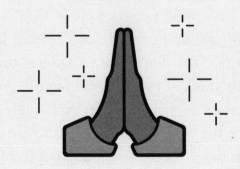

Are you ready for a break? Because I'm going to give you one. I've spent the last eleven actions telling you how to seize control of your day so you can give your life momentum. Now I'm going to tell you that control isn't everything. In fact, it's only part of the way your life moves forward every day. The other part involves a quantum force in the universe that operates independently of you and is beyond your ability to manage. I believe this power is completely good and always acts in your interest. It doesn't take a massive leap of faith to accept that it's out there, either. If you look at the events of your life, you'll have a hard time denying it.

Have I lost you? Just hear me out.

This universal force is not rooted in religion and doesn't concern itself with spirituality—unless you decide that seeing it either of those ways works for you. I call it "God" and "The Creator," but that's just my personal choice, rooted in beliefs that make sense to me. You don't have to name it anything if you don't want. Just think of the universal force of goodness as an autonomous energy, as mysterious yet explainable as the energy that sparked the Big Bang, and which furthers the growth of the universe to this day. It's that "something out there" that started life and has allowed it to continue for billions of years, despite all the ways humans have interfered. As my husband always says when he gives a lecture: We all believe in gravity even though we can't see it, right? Think of the universal force of goodness the same way. It's an energetic push through the unfolding events of life, with a reassuring inevitability that, even if things don't turn out the way we planned, there are lessons learned and happy outcomes in spite of it all.

Life Is Not Fair

Jennifer was a longtime therapist whose specialty was trauma. She'd counseled thousands of patients through unimaginably horrible situations, from sexual abuse to terminal illnesses to total financial ruin. In the weeks and months after 9/11, she worked onsite at the office of a Manhattan company that had relocated from one of the Twin Towers after terrorists destroyed them. A handful of people in her office had died, and those who survived were scarred for life by their terrifying escape, by the sound of bodies crashing to the pavement, by survivor's guilt, or by their lingering sense of uncertainty and loss. Jennifer was one of the first people many of them opened up to, letting all their trauma spill out.

Jennifer considered herself an optimist, and even though she saw people in the worst kinds of pain, she thought good counseling, support, and—when necessary—prescription drugs could help people through tough times. She also saw real resilience in many of her clients, and she knew that's what allowed them to persist—and sometimes thrive—despite what they'd been through. But when I brought up the notion of believing in a universal force of goodness, Jennifer was not having it.

"I had a patient who lost her three-year-old son to brain cancer, and you expect me to believe there's a force of goodness out there? If there is, she'd sure like to meet it."

Let me be clear here. I am absolutely *not* saying that everything happens for a reason. The death of that woman's son was not fair. It was soul-breaking. After seeing my mom's pain when my brother died, I cannot imagine anything worse than losing a child, especially an innocent baby. After my father and brother died, I had well-meaning people tell me that their deaths were part of God's plan or that they happened for some sort of purpose that wasn't my place to understand. That's not what I'm doing here.

What I am trying to get across is that life is not fair, but there are silver linings even in the worst of times. And there is a positive force guiding you all the time in the direction you are supposed to go that will lead to happiness. My dad's and brother's deaths were not in vain. Terrible things happen every single day, and I've experienced a good amount of them in my thirty-six years of life. But when I talk about a universal force of goodness, I am not explaining or defending them. I am simply saying that, through the tough stuff, the force that is the energy of life—call it a higher power, energy, or whatever you prefer—is still, on the whole, moving life in a constructive, forward direction.

You might find that silver lining inside yourself, as I did. I don't think I would have started my business if I hadn't lost so much that giving up a little more to follow my dreams didn't matter. I knew what it felt like to have nothing, so I figured, *Who cares if I make no money?* Or, that silver lining might exist in the unfolding events of the universe. The events of 9/11 were horrific, and they set in motion wars that continue to this day. But humanity has persisted because of its resilience. In fact, I'd argue that it's become resilient, in part, because of events like 9/11. Children have been born, people have fallen in love, new buildings have been built, and economies have recovered.

"What did you tell your client when her son died?" I asked Jennifer.

"Our conversations happened over a long period of time," she answered. "But the gist of what I said was that no matter what pain she faced, she had to try to choose goodness in her life. Happiness should be her goal because there was a lot of positive stuff in the world, too."

That "lot of positive stuff" is the universal force I'm talking about. Your greater power may not feel like it's present in every molecule of energy around you or in every second of time in the day, but it's there. You might as well recognize it. It's to your benefit to move toward it and allow it to give you the will to persevere even while you acknowledge that life is not always fair.

Most of us have heard the phrase "Without the rain, you can't appreciate the sun." The terrible things that happen in life are there just like stormy days that ruin your best-laid plans. You can't avoid them, and they inevitably will happen. But if they didn't occur, you'd be much less grateful for beautiful sunny days and you'd be less strong. In fact, you might take life's wonderful moments completely for granted.

I want you to believe in a universal force of goodness so that you can know that there is strength, humanity, and a sunny day even when life is at its most unfair. That goodness may not always be apparent—sometimes, after a week of rain, people forget what it feels like to have the sun on their faces—but that big ball of energy is behind those clouds. The bad and the good in life go

MOVE FORWARD EVERY DAY

There are several long-range medical studies that look at the connection between religion and longevity. One body of research published in the *Journal of the American Medical Association* determined that women who attended a religious service one or more times per week were 33 percent less likely to die during the sixteen-year follow-up period of the study than the subjects who didn't. A 2017 study published in *PLOS One* found that attending a religious service lowered subjects' stress response by a measurable degree and contributed to a 55 percent reduction in mortality during the eighteen years of the study.

Bear in mind that it may not be the religious aspect of going to a service that's correlated with a longer life. Church, temple, mass, community gatherings, and more draw people for many

hand in hand, but we should never, ever forget that there *is* positivity and that we should take action every single day to work toward it.

Nothing Is in Vain

In action eight, I talked about how I miscarried twins in late 2019. Every cell in my body mourned these babies, and my sense of loss was acute. But the entire process of loving then losing them expanded my life. In the midst of my anger and tears,

other reasons than worship. Many people attend religious services because of the community, the support, the value system, the mindfulness that comes with singing and praying, or the sense of purpose they feel by pulling themselves out of bed on a weekend morning. Some go because they like the free donuts and coffee, and some want free babysitting for an hour. It really doesn't matter as long as it lowers your stress response.

I think it's a great idea to attend or subscribe to almost any group situation that promotes personal and group well-being. Choose a yoga or Peloton class, even if it's online. Join a support group for whatever your bad habit or addiction is, or help lead a girl scout troop. The values these groups offer to your life may be your window into the concept of a universal force of goodness.

it wasn't always clear to me, but now I know that my grief was never, ever in vain. I learned something from it, and I moved forward—sometimes painfully—into a bigger and better life that has been impacted by those two precious souls.

That growth is part of the universal force of goodness. Even the absolute worst situations that happen in your life will ultimately give you a view toward something you can do better, be happier about, learn from, or grow with. Pain imparts real power and personal agency, even when you can't see it. The universal force of goodness stops you from falling apart and dying every single time something bad happens and inspires you to forge ahead, bruised but stronger.

I recently read about a man named Kevin Hines. Diagnosed with bipolar disorder when he was seventeen, Kevin was in constant emotional pain and began to fantasize about his own death. On September 24, 2000, when he was almost nineteen years old, he woke up in the morning and decided to end his life. He told his dad he loved him, wrote a suicide note, and took a bus to the edge of the Golden Gate Bridge in San Francisco, crying the whole way. He walked onto the bridge and paced back and forth from one end to the other. He passed tourists, police officers, and multiple call boxes with signs that urged anyone who was thinking of jumping to lift the receiver and ask for help. Kevin's mind didn't waver. He was fully committed to ending his life.

After about forty minutes, Kevin stopped and climbed over the rail, faced San Francisco Bay, and let go. As his body plummeted over the next four seconds, one thought entered his mind: that he'd

EVERYDAY WELLNESS | 275

made a terrible mistake, and that he wanted nothing more than to live. When he hit the water at 75 miles an hour, he went in feetfirst and at an angle, shattering several bones in his back. But he missed severing his spine by two millimeters, and he quickly bobbed to the surface and began swimming using only his arms.

Kevin had no idea at the time, but a woman on the bridge had seen him jump, and she'd called 911. A Coast Guard boat monitoring the bay spotted Kevin, and the captain pulled him on board before he could drown or die of hypothermia. It might as well have been a miracle; 98 to 99 percent of people who jump from the Golden Gate Bridge don't survive.

Kevin Hines now travels the world speaking about what happened to him, and while he doesn't describe his instantaneous, innate will to live in these terms, I think of it as the universal force of goodness. That energy told him the second he let go that life was better than death and that survival was absolutely, positively the right choice. That force mustered everything in its power to keep his spirit and body alive, like a flickering spark that pops and dances before it ignites into a full-fledged fire.

Kevin came very close to tragedy, but his immense suffering—before, during, and after his jump—wasn't in vain. Today, Hines says he uses small actions—from hugging a family member to waking up at the same time every morning—to give his mind and body a sense of comforting regularity and an occasional endorphin boost. He does the work to generate good, positive energy that keeps him speaking about mental illness and suicide and working as a mental health advocate. The intrinsic desire his body had to live that day, driven by a universal force of goodness, continues to allow him to keep putting good into the world every day.

MOVE FORWARD EVERY DAY

Sometimes it's helpful to think of the universal force of goodness as hope. Hope is much more than a feeling. It's a scientifically backed cognitive state that you establish by making goals, and is put in motion by expecting that you'll meet those goals. Hope holds the promise that you'll do your best work to achieve your dreams while accepting that other forces in the world at large are out of your hands.

Hope gives you optimism and strength and paves the way for resilience, and research shows that it lowers stress, reduces the risk for chronic disease, improves academic and athletic performance, enhances relationships, and more. So, why not welcome it into your life? Renowned psychologist and pioneer in the field of positive psychology Charles R. Snyder once said, *"A rainbow is a prism that sends shards of multicolored light in various directions. It lifts our spirits and makes us think of what is possible. Hope is the same—a personal rainbow of the mind."*

Pain and suffering are part of life. But there is also a larger, powerful force moving and connecting us in incredible ways. Whatever challenges we're facing, universal goodness shows you there's a larger lesson to be learned from everything. It doesn't matter if it's big (like a new baby), small (like a bad hair day), crushing (like a divorce), or seemingly insignificant, like the time a man named Noah skipped breakfast.

Noah was one of those people who's always there for everyone, often to the detriment of himself. One day, his little brother—who had a chronic inability to handle even the smallest issues without making a huge fuss—called him at 8 in the morning to ask him for a favor. Noah could tell he was frantic.

"I've got a problem with my car," his brother said, "and I'm hoping you can come over to help me fix it."

Noah usually worked out from 7 to 8, then made a protein smoothie immediately afterward. He loved his smoothie more than anything. It filled him up, settled the nausea he sometimes had after he worked out, and helped him focus his thoughts so he could start his day right. But when his brother called him, Noah tuned everything else out. He thought about asking him how urgent the issue was and whether it could be solved over the phone, but his relationship with his brother had been up and down for years, so he didn't want to rock the boat. He saw a problem, and he wanted to fix it, even if that meant putting his needs on the back burner. He threw on a pair of sweats, skipped making his smoothie, and walked out to his car so he could drive the twenty minutes to his brother's apartment.

278 | MARYRUTH GHIYAM

When he got there, his brother took ten minutes to put on his clothes. Then he took another ten minutes to find his keys, walk to his parking spot, and open up the hood. Even then, he wanted to talk more about his new girlfriend than he did about his car, and Noah pretty much had to force him to deal with the issue. After approximately ten seconds, it became clear what was going on.

"Well, looks like it's just a dead battery," his brother said. "Sorry. I guess I could have called AAA for that."

Hungry, impatient, and on edge because his blood sugar was so low, Noah flew into a rage and began yelling at his brother.

"I wasted an hour of my life for this? I thought it was an emergency!"

Noah stormed back to his car and tore out into traffic, narrowly missing hitting another car. When he finally pulled over and took a deep breath, he realized that all his problems that morning could have been avoided if he'd taken five minutes to eat breakfast. His head would have been clear, allowing him to figure out how urgent the issue was, his anxiety would have stayed low, and he never, ever would have screamed at his brother.

"I really regret my actions," Noah said, "but I don't think that explosion was in vain. It taught me something. You need to put on your own oxygen mask before you place one on someone else."

Noah had learned a lesson through an unpleasant situation. He didn't allow himself to become trapped in the past, full of regret, while his fight with his brother ate away at him. He understood nothing was in vain and that the confrontation unfolded so that he could stop being a victim. That, in turn, would make him a better brother. The universal force of goodness had pushed him ever so slightly into a direction where he could improve his life.

Let Go or Be Dragged

I've worked super hard to gain control over my life through routines and small actions that create structure. And while I have faith that a force greater than me is working toward good, I accept that much of my life is just not going to go the way I planned. In fact, I estimate that I'm disappointed, angered, or shocked by a full quarter of the outcomes in my life.

I know that sounds like too much, but stop and think about it. Consider all the things you do or go through in a twenty-four-hour period, from waking up in the morning to sitting in traffic to having a few tests done at the doctor. Many of these situations contain little bits of negativity—like if your doctor's running late or you have to fight your son to get him to brush his teeth at bedtime. These experiences may not be the end of the world, but they're not ideal. They leave a bad taste in your mouth, and no matter how much routine or structure you've put in place, that's just the way it is.

There is absolutely nothing you can do to control those little things. *Nothing.*

Much of the time, you have no say in the big events, either. When Ethan was first struggling to stand up, I did everything in my power to give him the best possible care, but it was up to him to take those first steps on his own. I can conceptualize the future of my company every day, and grow it by double digits every year, but I may still get an email that messes up my plans for a big product launch. No amount of planning or control reverses that disappointment.

I simply have to let go of the situation, and if I don't, I'll be dragged.

I *love* this phrase—let go or be dragged. People who thrive on planning—like me—are often reluctant to walk away from a losing battle or a situation that's spun into an impossibly difficult place. We think of accepting disappointments as a kind of defeat. But holding on to something you can't control will drag you along to the point of injury. Letting go, however, will give you the opportunity to stand up, dust yourself off, and turn to the good things in life that you have influence over. The whole world of possibility that's waiting for you is the universal force of goodness.

We often think of "let go or be dragged" in terms of personal relationships, but it can really deal with any toxic situation, like what Juan faced. Juan was a mild-mannered bar owner who'd been president of his condo board for a few years. While trying to cut costs so they could invest in a few capital projects, he and the rest of the board made the difficult decision to lay off two men on the building's maintenance staff. They knew this would help their bottom line and improve the building in the long term, but they also understood it would be viewed negatively by some of the residents. People loved these staff members and thought of them as family.

Unfortunately, the backlash against the board was much worse than they expected. A small group of residents banded together and picketed the next board meeting. Someone called the local news, and a story ran the next night. A movement formed around the two fired maintenance men, and Juan was urged by the rest of the board to resign so they could save face.

Months later, Juan was still traumatized by the situation and couldn't let it go. He fumed about it, posted about it on Facebook, texted the neighbors who were on his side, and tried to rally people together to undo what he perceived to be all the damage that had been done to the condo—not to mention his reputation. *I took the fall for everyone,* he thought. *I have to prove that I didn't do anything wrong.* But the other residents were exhausted by the situation. There had been a problem, a solution had been found, and now they wanted to move on with their lives. No one wanted their building to be a war zone.

Juan was in a toxic stranglehold with a situation that was beyond his control. No matter what he did, his best efforts to drum up opposition to the people who'd punished him—and drum up support for himself—were just not going to materialize as he hoped. Juan needed to step back and let go. And, if he didn't, he was going to be dragged.

After about two weeks of not sending angry texts to friends and not drafting angry responses to the posts that showed up on

MOVE FORWARD EVERY DAY

You're doing the twelve actions to the best of your ability every single day. They're empowering you, making you more self-aware, and improving your body, mind, and spirit in subtle ways that really add up. Your life is moving forward every day, and you should be super proud of that. Congratulations from the bottom of my heart.

The self-care my book introduces to you is essential to better living, but we are all part of the collective, and we have to help each other if we want *the world* to move forward. While you're taking care of yourself, don't forget to help others. Giving back prevents depression, lowers high blood pressure, unifies families, builds a community, and so much more. Charitable giving—whether it's time, money, or living by example—is as essential to your self-care routine as getting exercise or sleeping at least seven hours. Make it part of your routine every day you're able.

There's a universal force of goodness in the world, and you are a part of it.

the condo's Facebook group, Juan started to feel a little lighter. His friends appreciated that he wasn't always talking about how upset he was, and his wife was relieved to see him take interest in the activities he used to love. After a month, Juan didn't tense up as much when he walked into the lobby. One day, he noticed that the flowers outside the building looked nice, and he remembered that he'd urged the landscapers to plant them. Instead of feeling bitter, he felt good.

All this time, there had been a force of goodness that was waiting to move him into a more optimistic, happy place in his life, yet he was holding on to his negative, painful feelings and his complete inability to control things. For Juan, letting go wasn't a failure. It was a show of strength for himself and his position in life. When he wasn't toxic any longer, maybe he could return to the issue and seek change. But, first, he needed to look for the positive.

In your life, you have to create a balance between that which you can control and that which you can't. I want you to head down a road in your life where you encounter only green lights. There were no green lights for Juan when it came to his condo board, so he had to be aware of the red lights, then walk away. In life, sometimes we need to let go and sometimes we need to push forward and move mountains to get what we want. Just pay attention, judge and act to the best of your ability, and know there is a force guiding you. Whether or not you can control what life hands you, remember that there's a world of good energy waiting for you no matter what.

Conclusion

· ·

About a month after I finished writing this book, I gave birth to my twins. In the span of a few minutes, I went from a mother of two to a mother of four. That's double the mouths to feed. Double the times startled awake during the night. Double the hard-to-understand, superficially irrational needs and wants that pull parents away from their jobs, routines, and personal lives.

I'm not going to lie to you. The first few months were *hard*. Having four children in three years and four months while working on my business was so difficult. But, like so many new parents lost in the confusion and wonder of new parenting, I made a conscious decision to look at my wildly changed life differently. I now had double the possibilities for my children to change the world. Double the hope for a brighter future—for me, my family, and everyone around us. Double the opportunity to be a loving, strong example to help them grow into generous, capable citizens of the world.

When I looked at those two tiny, new faces—Jacob and Grace—I forced myself to think about the future even though the present seemed incredibly intense. Then I embraced one of the central messages of this book: self-awareness. I said as kindly to myself as possible: *MaryRuth, I know this is the hardest thing you've ever done, but it's also the most important. You are the mother of these babies and you are their world. Be the best you can for them.* I made being a good wife and mother my goal, as well as taking care of my employees and customers. Then I worked backward, asking myself how I could get there. The answer lay entirely within how I conducted myself within each twenty-four-hour period.

I was barely holding myself together sometimes. The memory of driving Ethan half an hour to and from physical therapy every single day when Elliot was six weeks old seemed like a piece of cake. Now I was pumping breast milk for two babies, working full time on my business, and I had an entire pumping station in my office devoted to feeding them. I'd set up a table with thirty bottles on it, and I rotated through all of them in a few days. The only thing that could prevent me from feeling overwhelmed every day was the structure and routine that grounded me, then prepared me to spring into action so I could move forward. My twelve actions were where I started that process each and every day.

Some days I could only work through one or two of them, and that was okay. You may go a week or a month without doing any, and that's also fine. Just know that they're there for you. My program is a lifelong journey through many seasons, and some of those times are chaos. Don't stress; just return to the twelve actions when you can. They'll offer you energy and momentum whatever your situation—positive or negative.

Routine and organization grant you incredible power, and the structure you build within each day will give you the freedom to be truly happy. If you take away anything from this book, I want you to know that happiness and satisfaction are entirely within your reach. You can make it there just by chewing your food until it's liquid, letting the sun wash over you for fifteen minutes, or by stretching while you're stuck on a conference call. Minute by minute, day by day, you'll inch forward and, before you know it, those micro changes will add up and become life changing.

Acknowledgments

. . . .

God: I truly believe that God always wants the best for each one of us, and everything that happens to us is God gently and lovingly moving us forward every single day in our lives.

My dad, Richard: You passed away suddenly when I was twelve years old. It is incredible how much you molded me in just twelve years. Your love was always so strong, and I remember watching you make your to-do lists (yellow legal pads and red pen). That is something I have carried with me my entire life that has moved me forward. Love you.

My mom, Colleen: We have been through everything together and have been by each other's side for all of it. You are the one and only person who truly showed me how to move forward every day. I love you.

My brother, Daniel: You passed away suddenly when you were seventeen years old. I carry the love between us in my heart and in my mind every single day. No one could make me laugh harder. Your life was not in vain, and so much of my ability to help other people and love other people has to do with losing you. I love you always.

My husband, David: We were born on the same day in the same year, February 11, 1984, two hours and twenty-four minutes apart. Thank you for all of your love and for giving our family the most beautiful life ever. I love you, David.

Ethan, Elliot, Jacob, and Grace: Thank you for making me a mom and showing me how to be the best version of myself. It is with utter and complete joy that I watch you grow up into the people you are meant to become. I am always here for you, and I love you with my whole heart.

Shirin and Mike: Thank you for being the best mother- and father-in-law a person could want. Thank you for your unconditional love and for raising David to be so loving as well.

Dan and Sanam: Thank you for being so loving. I feel blessed that you are my brother- and sister-in-law. You are always there for us.

Peter McGuigan and Sarah Durand: To my book agent, Peter, and our writer, Sarah. You are the greatest people to work with and a powerful team. I feel so lucky to have done this book with you both.

Judith Curr, Gideon Weil, Sam Tatum, Courtney Nobile, Aly Mostel, Julia Kent, and the HarperOne team: I will always remember the day in February 2020 that I first met Judith, Gideon, Courtney, and your team. Thank you for believing in the power of this book and its ability to help people all over the world live healthier lives.

Kaitlan Mattern: To our very first MaryRuth Organics employee. I respect you so much for all the hard work that you do every single day to help all of our customers live healthier lives. Your hard work and leadership of our entire team is truly inspirational to everyone around you. Thank you for everything.

Crystal Chow: To one of our very talented graphic designers on our team. Thank you for the most beautiful images for this book. The infographic for "The Art of Health for Busy People" is a tool that helps people live a healthier life every single day! Your work is truly appreciated on so many levels by everyone.

MRO Team: To the entire MaryRuth Organics team—for me to work with such incredible people is one of the greatest things in my life! I feel that our collective effort day in and day out has helped millions of people to live healthier lives. Thank you for your dedication and your heart!

To Maria, Blanca, Edith, Mercy, Camila, and Georgina: Thank you for all of your daily support and true care. You make a powerful team.

To our customers and our readers: Thank you for supporting our brand and for reading this book! I hope that each person who reads this book will gain a positive momentum in their own life to move forward every day toward what makes them healthy and happy!

Sources

Action One

Shen, Run, Biao Wang, Maria G. Giribaldi, Janelle Ayres, John B. Thomas, and Marc Montminy. "Neuronal Energy-Sensing Pathway Promotes Energy Balance by Modulating Disease Tolerance." *Proceedings of the National Academy of Sciences* 113, no. 23 (June 7, 2016): E3307–E3314.

Action Two

Higgs, Suzanne, and Alison Jones. "Corrigendum to 'Prolonged Chewing at Lunch Decreases Later Snack Intake.'" *Appetite* 116 (September 1, 2017): 616.

Action Three

Hosseinlou, Abdollah, Saeed Khamnei, and Masumeh Zamanlu. "The Effect of Water Temperature and Voluntary Drinking on the Post Rehydration Sweating." *International Journal of Clinical and Experimental Medicine* 6, no. 8 (September 1, 2013): 683–87.

Maughan, Ronald J., Phillip Watson, Philip AA Cordery, Neil P. Walsh, Samuel J. Oliver, Alberto Dolci, Nidia Rodriguez-Sanchez, and Stuart D. R. Galloway. "A Randomized Trial to Assess the Potential of Different Beverages to Affect Hydration Status: Development of a Beverage Hydration Index." *The American Journal of Clinical Nutrition* 103, no. 3 (March 2016): 717–23.

Pizzorno, Joseph. "Acidosis: An Old Idea Validated by New Research." *Integrative Medicine* 14, no. 1 (2015): 8–12.

Pross, Nathalie, Agnès Demazières, Nicolas Girard, Romain Barnouin, Déborah Metzger, Alexis Klein, Erica Perrier, and Isabelle Guelinckx. "Effects of Changes in Water Intake on Mood of High and Low Drinkers." *PLOS One* 9, no. 4 (April 11, 2014): e94754. doi:10.1371/journal.pone.0094754.

Action Four

Kitahara, Cari M., et al. "Association Between Class III Obesity (BMI of 40–59 kg/m^2) and Mortality: A Pooled Analysis of 20 Prospective Studies." *PLOS Medicine* (July 8, 2014). https://doi.org/10.1371/journal.pmed.1001673.

Turek, Fred W., et al. "Obesity and Metabolic Syndrome in Circadian Clock Mutant Mice." *Science* 308, no. 5724 (2005): 1043–5.

Action Five

Spoor, Kesha Dorsey, and Hala Madanat. "Relationship Between Body Image Discrepancy and Intuitive Eating." *International Quarterly of Community Health Education* 36, no. 3 (April 2016): 189–97.

Vohs, Kathleen D., Joseph P. Redden, and Ryan Rahinel. "Physical Order Produces Healthy Choices, Generosity, and Conventionality, Whereas Disorder Produces Creativity." *Psychological Science* 24, no. 9 (2013): 1860–7.

Action Six

Georgetown University Medical Center. "Sunlight Offers Surprise Benefit: It Energizes Infection Fighting T Cells." *ScienceDaily* (December 20, 2016). www.sciencedaily.com/releases/2016/12/161220094633.htm.

Heiland, Teresa L., Robert Rovetti, and Jan Dunn. "Effects of Visual, Auditory, and Kinesthetic Imagery Interventions on Dancers' Plié Arabesques." *Journal of Imagery Research in Sport and Physical Activity* 7, no. 1 (January 2012).

Hossein-nezhad, Arash, and Michael F. Holick. "Vitamin D for Health: A Global Perspective." *Mayo Clinic Proceedings* 88, no. 7 (2013): 720–55.

Mead, M. Nathaniel. "Benefits of Sunlight: a Bright Spot for Human Health." *Environmental Health Perspectives* 116, no. 4 (2008): A160–67.

Uppsala University. "Plenty of Daytime Light May Reduce Effects of Blue Light Screens on Sleep." *NeuroscienceNews* (August 10, 2016). https://neuroscience news.com/daytime-light-blue-screen-sleep-4817.

Action Seven

Van Dongen, Hans P. A., Greg Maislin, Janet M. Mullington, and David F. Dinges. "The Cumulative Cost of Additional Wakefulness: Dose-Response Effects on Neurobehavioral Functions and Sleep Physiology from Chronic Sleep Restriction and Total Sleep Deprivation." *Sleep* (March 15, 2003): 117–26.

Action Eight

Simic, L., N. Sarabon, and G. Markovic. "Does Pre-Exercise Static Stretching Inhibit Maximal Muscular Performance? A Meta-Analytical Review." *Scandinavian Journal of Medicine & Science in Sports* 23, no. 2 (2013): 131–48.

Action Nine

Gonzalez, Javier T., Rachel C. Veasey, Penny L. S. Rumbold, and Emma J. Stevenson. "Breakfast and Exercise Contingently Affect Postprandial Metabolism and Energy Balance in Physically Active Males." *British Journal of Nutrition* 110, no. 4 (August 2013): 721–32.

Loprinzi, Paul D., and Bradley J. Cardinal. "Association Between Objectively-Measured Physical Activity and Sleep, NHANES 2005–2006." *Mental Health and Physical Activity* 4, no. 2 (December 2011): 65–69.

Puetz, Timothy W., Sara S. Flowers, and Patrick J. O'Connor. "A Randomized Controlled Trial of the Effect of Aerobic Exercise Training on Feelings of Energy and Fatigue in Sedentary Young Adults with Persistent Fatigue." *Psychotherapy and Psychosomatics* 77, no. 3 (2008): 167–74.

Sharma, Ashish, Vishal Madaan, and Frederick D. Petty. "Exercise for Mental Health." *Primary Care Companion to the Journal of Clinical Psychiatry* 8, no. 2 (2006): 106.

Action Ten

Koelsch, Stefan, Julian Fuermetz, Ulrich Sack, Katrin Bauer, Maximilian Hohenadel, Martin Wiegel, Udo X. Kaisers, and Wolfgang Heinke. "Effects of Music Listening on Cortisol Levels and Propofol Consumption During Spinal Anesthesia." *Frontiers in Psychology* 2, no. 58 (April 5, 2011). doi:10.3389/fpsyg.2011.00058.

Action Eleven

Rosenbaum, Jerrold F., and Jennifer M. Covino. "Stress and Resilience: Implications for Depression and Anxiety." *Medscape* (December 29, 2005).